small
changes
BIG
results

small changes
BIG
results

A Wellness Plan with 65 Recipes for a Healthy, Balanced Life Full of Flavor

Revised and Updated

ellie krieger

with kelly james-enger

Clarkson Potter/Publishers
New York

Published in the United States by Clarkson Potter/Publishers,
an imprint of the Crown Publishing Group, a division of Random House, Inc., New York.
www.crownpublishing.com
www.clarksonpotter.com

CLARKSON POTTER is a trademark and POTTER with colophon
is a registered trademark of Random House, Inc.

Originally published in the United States in different form by Clarkson Potter/Publishers,
an imprint of the Crown Publishing Group, a division of Random House, Inc., New York, in 2005.

Grateful acknowledgment is made to Center for Science in the Public Interest for permission to
reprint an excerpt from *Nutrition Action Healthletter*. Copyright © 2004 by CSPI. Reprinted by
permission of Center for Science in the Public Interest, 1975 Connecticut Ave., NW, Suite 300,
Washington, DC, 20009-5728.

Library of Congress Cataloging-in-Publication Data
First Revised Edition
Krieger, Ellie.
  Small changes, big results / Ellie Krieger with Kelly James-Enger. —Revised and updated.
  1. Health.   2. Physical fitness.   3. Nutrition.   I. James-Enger, Kelly.   II. Title.
  RA776.K6986 2012
  613—dc23   2012017628

ISBN 978-0-307-98557-6
eISBN 978-0-307-98558-3

Printed in the United States of America

Book design by Ashley Tucker
Illustrations by Meredith Noyes
Cover design by Rae Ann Spitzenberger
Cover photography © Melanie Acevedo

10 9 8 7 6 5 4 3 2 1

First Revised Edition

for **Thom** & **Isabella**

contents

recipes

preface

Two things sum up my motivation to revise this book: Greek yogurt and iPods. When *Small Changes, Big Results* was first published in 2005, Greek yogurt was available only in specialty stores, so the recipes that called for it included instructions to make it yourself. And, iPods were just beginning to gain a foothold as a consumer staple. It was the era of the Walkman. (Remember those?) There were no apps or smart phones, and few people had heard of quinoa.

But while the world has changed remarkably since the book's original publication, the basic plan I put forth then has stood the test of time. The path of small changes with a whole-life approach of eating well, getting fit, and feeling good continues to be backed by science as a sound way to a healthy, happy life. On top of that I now have the testimonials of a multitude of people who have transformed their lives using this plan.

What's more, the Usually/Sometimes/Rarely food philosophy, which I originally laid out in the first edition, has proved a guiding force for my work over the years and has been the foundation of the all recipes I developed for my Food Network show *Healthy Appetite* and for my award-winning cookbooks.

So what's new here? Besides the inclusion of iPods and Greek yogurt, lots. First of all, there are many more recipes—65 in all—to help make your weekly "Eating Well" changes more delicious and easier than ever. I have also updated the food sections to reflect the latest science and new options at the grocery store. For example, we now know sugar is worse for you and coffee and coconut are better for you than we once thought. We know we need more vitamin D and that spices contain powerful antioxidants. Besides refreshing the information on those items, I give you the scoop on hot topics like agave, stevia, gluten, and local eating. And I incorporate more foods like quinoa and edamame, which were once hard to find but are now in most stores.

On the fitness front, I address popular classes like Zumba and yoga and guide you to websites and apps that can help you stay on track with the weekly changes and make an active life more accessible. The Feeling Good sections now include ways to balance new technology in your life, from finding ways to "unplug" to making the most of social media.

What you'll find here is a fresh, modern approach to a plan that has tried-and-true benefits. I passionately believe in *Small Changes, Big Results*, and I am thrilled to have been able to update it here to continue to inspire healthy living for years to come.

introduction

Imagine yourself the best person you can be. You wake up each morning energized, feeling comfortable and confident in your body, moving with ease, and standing tall. Your life is full and exciting, yet you are grounded with a sense of balance. You are able to think fast and flow with life's challenges. You are surrounded by people you love, supported by them, and supporting them in turn. And you know you are doing what you can to live a longer, healthier life.

You may feel this ideal is unattainable at times. But let me tell you something: you can be that person (or at least come close—you are human, after all!). All you have to do is make some small changes.

Most people *want* to look better, feel better, and live happier, more fulfilling lives. They may be motivated to make a change, but they're not sure what to do first—or they're overwhelmed by the idea of overhauling their entire lives. They get stuck before they even begin.

The problem isn't lack of information—there's more data about nutrition, fitness, and wellness available than ever before. In fact, we've instead become victims of information overload. Should you cut out red meat from your diet or keep it in? Increase protein intake or eliminate carbs? Exercise seven days a week or only three? Lift weights or do yoga? We are bombarded by information every day, and it's nearly impossible to sort out what's helpful and valuable from some of the get-thin-quick schemes that almost never work.

Many people want to change the way they eat and the way they treat their bodies, but they underestimate how multifaceted this kind of transformation can be. Or they bite off more than they can chew and try to change *everything* all at once. The problem is that they may not have the tools they need to change their lifestyle, or they become overwhelmed by trying to do too much too soon.

Does this sound familiar? Well, I'm here to help you, and I've got good news: you *don't* have to overhaul your entire lifestyle or subject yourself to the latest fad diet. Making *small* changes is the key to transforming your life. By making small changes in your diet, activity level, and lifestyle, you can change the way you eat, move, and feel—without having to suffer, without needing expensive equipment or special foods, and without feeling overwhelmed.

I take a three-pronged approach. I'm a dietitian and professional cook, but my focus is on more than just food and nutrition. **I look at nutrition, fitness, and wellness as a three-legged stool**. Each leg supports the others, and all are necessary for a balanced life.

In the chapters that follow, you'll learn how to make small changes in these three areas of your life. You'll be introduced to my 12-Week Wellness Plan, which gives you all the tools you need, including 65 recipes, to help you change your life. Each week sets out specific small changes in the way you eat, the way you move, and the way you live and explains how to make the change as well as why it will benefit you. By progressing in bite-size chunks and building on what you did before, you'll find that eating, exercising, and living more healthfully is easier, and more delicious than you thought.

eating well

When most people think about eating better or losing weight, they think about how restrictive they need to be and what to say *no* to. When you focus on what you can't have, it's no wonder you feel deprived and irritable! I take the opposite approach and **concentrate on what you can say yes to**.

Sure, there are foods you have to cut back on if you want to lose weight. Most of us can't down pizza and milk shakes all day without the extra calories showing up on our tummies or thighs. But food is not an enemy. Food is a wonderful, delicious, sensuous part of life, and it doesn't have to stop being so just because you're eating healthfully.

I help people discover all the great foods they can say yes to. When I talk about the "ideal" diet, I frame it in terms of what types of foods to eat rather than what foods to avoid. An ideal diet provides you with a wide variety of nutritious, delicious foods that you enjoy. It's a diet you can maintain because you like what you're eating, not a diet you have to force yourself to stick to. (See Appendix B on page 292 for a sample week's healthy—and delicious—ideal diet.)

Don't confuse an "ideal" diet with a "perfect" diet. There's no such thing as a perfect diet! In fact, people who constantly strive for the "perfect" diet often become obsessive about food and eating, which can be just as unhealthy and destructive as ignoring the way you eat.

In my wellness plan, there are no forbidden foods, but there are foods that you should eat rarely or occasionally. You don't have to vow that you'll never have chocolate cake again in order to make useful changes in your eating patterns. Instead of grouping foods and our eating patterns associated with them into extreme categories—all or nothing, good or bad—I find it helps to categorize foods into three groups:

- **usually**—foods you should base your diet on, and the foods you can freely say yes to. Fruits, vegetables, whole grains, legumes, nuts, lean proteins, healthy oils, and low-fat dairy products are all Usually foods.

- **sometimes**—foods you can sometimes say yes to, like refined grains, higher-fat meats, and sugary foods.

- **rarely**—foods that you should only rarely say yes to—junk food, candy, fatty meats, and high-fat desserts. Yes, they can still be a part of a healthy diet. But they should be indulgences, not for every day.

The nutritional component of my 12-Week Wellness Plan doesn't force you to suddenly change the way you're currently eating. Instead, you'll focus on one skill at a time, from learning the optimal timing for your meals to gradually incorporating the best foods into your life—the foods that will help keep you slim, healthy, and energized. There are 65 recipes; plus all the tips along the way will give you all the tools you need to change successfully.

Finally, I offer you a way of eating, *not* a diet. As I see it, a diet is something you go on until you lose weight and then you go off it. It is a losing (or should I say regaining?) mentality. To lose weight for good and to be optimally healthy, you need to make changes you can live with. My plan allows you to make small changes in the way you're eating now that will add up to better nutrition, more energy, and weight loss over the long haul.

getting fit

Eating well is only one part of the picture. You also have to be physically active to stay slim, feel your best, and live healthier. Many people moan and groan when I say this, because they have forgotten how good it actually feels to move with regularity.

Ask any dedicated exerciser why he or she does it, and answers will vary. "It helps me maintain my weight." "I can leave the stressors of the day behind at the gym." "Exercise gives me more energy." "It helps keep me healthy." But one of the most common reasons is a simple one—"It makes me feel good."

the usually/sometimes/rarely food lists

usually
These foods should be the backbone of your daily diet. Aim to get most of your daily servings from this group.

vegetables
- Any vegetable—fresh, frozen, or low-sodium canned (but not fried or in cream sauces)

fruits
- Fruit—fresh, frozen (unsweetened), or canned in natural juice (not sweetened syrup)

whole grains and starchy vegetables
- Whole-grain bread, whole-grain rolls, whole wheat bagels
- Whole-grain, low-sugar cold breakfast cereals (Shredded Wheat, Bran Flakes, Cheerios, etc.)
- Whole-grain, low-sugar hot breakfast cereals (oatmeal, Wheatena, brown rice cereal, etc.)
- Whole-grain, low-fat crackers (Wasa Crispbread)
- Whole-grain pasta, brown rice, whole wheat couscous, bulgur, quinoa, buckwheat
- Whole wheat or corn tortillas
- Whole wheat pretzels, air-popped popcorn
- Potatoes, sweet potatoes, corn

seafood, meat, poultry, and eggs
- Seafood—any fish or shellfish not on the Sometimes or Rarely list. (Women who are pregnant, may become pregnant, or are nursing, and small children should eat up to 12 ounces of fish a week total.)
- Poultry—turkey breast, lean or extra-lean ground turkey, skinless chicken breast
- Beef—eye of round, top sirloin, top loin (strip) steak, 95% lean ground beef
- Pork—tenderloin, loin, extra-lean ham
- Game meats—venison, ostrich, buffalo
- Egg whites

beans, soy, nuts, and seeds
- Any beans, lentils, black-eyed peas, split peas, chickpeas
- Soy—soy milk, tofu, tempeh, miso
- Nuts—walnuts, almonds, pistachios, hazelnuts, pecans, macadamia nuts, peanuts
- Seeds—pumpkin seeds, sunflower seeds, sesame seeds, flaxseed
- Peanut butter, almond butter, other nut butters

low-fat dairy
- Skim and 1% low-fat milk
- Low-fat plain yogurt
- Low-fat cottage cheese
- Low-fat buttermilk

healthy fats and oils
- Olive oil, flaxseed oil, canola oil, peanut oil, safflower oil, walnut oil

sometimes
These foods are more processed, contain more added sugar, and/or more saturated fat and cholesterol than those on the Usually list, but they are fine to include in your diet in moderation. Aim to have no more than three servings from this list per day.

vegetables
- Coleslaw and other vegetable salads with creamy dressings
- Vegetables with cream sauces (creamed spinach)
- Vegetable juice

fruits
- Coconut
- 100% fruit juice

grains and starchy vegetables
- Breads, rolls, and bagels made with refined (white) flour
- Cold cereals that are not whole-grain
- Crackers that are not whole-grain
- Biscuits, pancakes, waffles
- White rice, regular pasta
- Granola bars, reduced-calorie muffins
- Baked chips

seafood, meat, poultry, and eggs
- Seafood—bluefish, North American lobster, orange roughy, fresh tuna, canned albacore/white tuna. (Women who are pregnant, may become pregnant, or are nursing, and small children should limit these fish to no more than 6 ounces of the 12 ounces total per week.)
- Poultry—chicken breast with skin, chicken leg with skin, skinless chicken thigh, skinless duck breast, poultry sausage
- Beef—top round, chuck shoulder pot roast, brisket (flat half) tenderloin, flank steak, T-bone steak (all trimmed of fat), 90% lean ground beef
- Lamb—sirloin, shank, shoulder
- Pork—Canadian bacon, regular ham
- Whole eggs

dairy
- Whole milk
- Full-fat cottage cheese
- Full-fat and/or heavily sweetened yogurt
- Part-skim mozzarella and ricotta cheeses
- Reduced-fat sour cream, reduced-fat cream cheese

fats
- "Vegetable" oil, corn oil, sesame oil, grapeseed oil
- Mayonnaise

sweets
- Honey, maple syrup, molasses, agave
- High-quality dark chocolate
- Lower-calorie cookies and cakes, such as fig bars, gingersnaps, graham crackers, biscotti, angel food cake
- Frozen yogurt, ice milk, fruit bars, fruit sorbets

continues ›››

rarely

These foods are highly processed and/or have a lot of saturated fat, trans fat, and refined sugar. Aim for five servings or fewer from this list per week.

vegetables
- Fried or battered and fried vegetables

fruits
- Fruit "drinks" or "cocktails"
- Fruit canned in syrup

grains and starchy vegetables
- Packaged baked goods and crackers made with hydrogenated or partially hydrogenated vegetable oil (avoid entirely or strictly limit)
- Heavily sweetened cold cereals and bars
- Fried chips
- French fries, fried potatoes
- Full-fat muffins made with white flour

seafood, meat, and poultry
- Seafood—king mackerel, shark, swordfish, tilefish (Strictly limit. Women who are pregnant, may become pregnant, or are nursing, and small children should avoid these fish entirely.)
- Poultry—Chicken thigh or wing, with skin, 85% lean ground turkey, chicken or duck liver
- Beef—85% lean ground beef, corned beef, short ribs, prime rib, calf's liver
- Pork—pork ribs, pork butt, pork shoulder
- Processed meats—hot dogs, bologna, salami, regular sausage, bacon

dairy
- Full-fat cheeses
- Heavy cream, whipped cream
- Full-fat sour cream
- Crème fraîche
- Cream cheese

fats
- Butter
- Coconut oil
- Lard
- Margarine and vegetable shortening (avoid entirely unless trans fat–free)

sweets
- Granulated/white sugar, brown sugar
- Candy—most commercial candy bars
- Pies, cakes, cookies, doughnuts, pastries
- Ice cream

When you're in good physical shape, activity *does* feel good. Dancers, runners, yoga devotees, weight lifters, and dedicated walkers all experience a mental and physical lift from exercise. This feeling, sometimes called a runner's high, creates an emotional boost and a positive sense of well-being.

Yet you needn't be a dedicated athlete to experience this joy of movement. Watch children playing: they run for the fun of it, jump in the air because it feels good. Somewhere between early childhood and teenage years, though, most of us begin to lose the spontaneous joy of this experience and settle down to a lifetime of using our bodies only when we need them, which in our push-button, technology-driven world isn't very often.

But our bodies are meant to move! Just because modern life has become more sedentary doesn't mean we have to be. When exercise is a healthy habit, you'll notice a difference. You'll feel more energetic, more alert, and more alive. Regular exercise strengthens your immune system, builds stronger muscles and bones, and improves your cardiovascular health, reducing your risk of heart attacks and a slew of other conditions. It changes the way your body looks and the way you feel about your body—not just your physical appearance but your capabilities, as well. It reduces anxiety, eases depression, and elevates mood.

If you haven't been in good physical shape since grade school, it can be tough getting started. I've found that most people have similar excuses (oops, I mean "reasons") when it comes to not exercising. "I don't have time!" is the number one reason; "I'm too tired" follows close on its heels. I think, though, that a major obstacle is that people start out and usually don't exercise regularly enough or long enough for it to begin to feel good to them. They never get over the initial hump to make exercise a part of their lives.

Many people begin aggressively and then find that the inevitable soreness and fatigue provides them with the perfect excuse they need to give up exercise . . . until next year's New Year's resolutions roll around. But if you start slowly and proceed gradually, you begin to see and feel the results, and those results become your incentive to make activity a priority. Let me tell you, I am not always gung-ho to work out. I sometimes have to drag myself to the gym or out for a walk. But no matter how much I'd rather stay in bed, knowing from experience how a little exercise brings me to life and how it keeps me feeling good in my jeans somehow gets me going.

Even if you've been a dedicated couch potato for as long as you can remember, I'll help you make exercise happen in your own life. The fitness component of the 12-Week Wellness Plan is easy, doable, accessible, and well-rounded. It includes all three elements of a comprehensive fitness program—strength, flexibility, and cardiovascular exercise.

I've made things easy by providing a program designed for anyone who hasn't exercised before or is coming back to working out after a long period of inactivity. (But, as with any exercise program, please get your doctor's okay before you start.) And if you're a regular exerciser, you can use this framework and tweak it to make it challenging enough for you, as well.

Best of all, you can start at a level that's well within reach and build on what you've done before so that, as your body becomes fitter, you're ready for each new step and challenge as the weeks go by. Moving more isn't only about exercising—it's about beginning to make movement a part of your life. I'll help you change your mind-set and your approach so that you're leading an active life.

feeling good

The third component of the wellness program is often overlooked by fitness-minded people. They realize it is important to eat better and move their bodies more, but they're surprised when I tell them there is one more key factor—to examine their lives to determine the biggest stressors, and figure out ways to reduce or eliminate them.

You can eat well and exercise regularly, but if you ignore your mental health and emotional well-being, you won't feel good. Learning how to manage stress is an integral part of this program, as is mindfulness, which I'll discuss in a moment.

While stress has as many definitions as there are individuals, in medical terms it describes your body's response to events or actions that it perceives as threatening. You may have heard of the "fight or flight" response: our ancestors had to be physiologically equipped to deal with stressors such as encountering a predator. When they sensed fear, their breathing and heart rate increased, and their heart pumped more blood to their muscles to prepare the body to respond. Adrenaline and other hormones were produced to prepare the person to either battle the predator or flee. After the initial threat was encountered, the body's systems would return to normal.

Today, though we're unlikely to run into a saber-toothed tiger on the commute to work, our bodies are still programmed the same way. Events that scare or worry or anger us produce this stress response, where breathing becomes faster and shallower, heart rate and blood pressure increase, and stress hormones like adrenaline and cortisol surge. The problem is that stress for many people becomes chronic, or constant, which affects us both physically and emotionally.

I'll show you how to reduce stress in your day-to-day life. Beating daily stress can have a significant effect on your eating habits, too. Stress often compels people to skip meals, overeat, and/or eat lots of sugary, fatty foods. Also, researchers are finding that being subject to chronic stress affects hormones that make you more likely to gain weight around your middle and may make it harder to shed pounds.

That's one of the reasons I want you to do more than look at *what* you put into your body and do to your body. I want you to reflect on how you cope with stress. For example, when I was in private practice, I worked with a lot of people who were emotional eaters—they turned to food when they were angry, upset, lonely, depressed, or anxious. As their nutritionist, I helped them cope with stress and other difficult feelings, and that helped with their eating, as well. I'm not a psychologist, but sometimes emotional issues are what I call connecting points between nutrition, fitness, and wellness. You're overeating because you're stressed, and you rely on food to calm your nerves. When you learn how to manage your stress better, you also eat better; if you can cope with some of those underlying reasons, it frees you up to look at food a different way.

But the third part of my program is about more than managing stress, too. It's about becoming more aware of your life, what makes you happy, and taking steps to enhance your happiness. Wellness is about nurturing yourself and your relationships, because ultimately that's one of the keys to your health and happiness. Self-esteem, adequate sleep, and supportive, happy relationships contribute to health just as much as eating right and exercising. Giving your body a chance to rest and repair, maintaining good relationships—a sense of connectedness in your life—and having a sense of purpose all help you stay healthy, maintain your weight, and prevent disease just as exercise and eating well do.

My plan has three elements—nutrition, fitness, and lifestyle—that are all interconnected. Becoming more emotionally healthy and reducing stress will make it easier for you to make smarter food choices and make you more likely to stick with your fitness routine. And when you work out regularly, you feel better about yourself and about your body, which helps with your overall happiness—and makes you more likely to want to eat better because you want to give your body the fuel it needs. Each element supports the others.

If you're unhappy with the shape of your body or the size of your thighs, it's natural to turn to a diet or exercise program in search of the results you want. But true fitness comes from integrating body, mind, and spirit. If you focus only on your external self, your life will feel empty. **It's only by honoring your inner self and developing a healthy balance that you'll feel truly fulfilled.**

how to use this book

This book is designed to walk you through small changes over the space of 12 weeks. Each week I provide small, specific action steps in the three core wellness areas—Eating Well, Getting Fit, and Feeling Good—along with all the tools you need to accomplish those steps.

While each of the 12 weeks' changes are critical to the Eating Well and Getting Fit elements, the core of the Feeling Good program is established once you reach the halfway point, after the first six weeks. After that point, the Feeling Good action steps enhance the core plan but are less essential, so I have offered them as optional. I'd like you to try several of them, but I don't want you to feel overwhelmed by having to do them all. If you incorporate the Feeling Good action steps of the first six weeks, you'll have a solid, effective lifestyle plan in place. The changes in the weeks that follow are designed to further enrich your life. I suggest you try at least three of the Feeling Good changes in Weeks 7 through 12.

That said, the way you use this book is completely up to you, and I encourage you to personalize your experience with it. You can read through it all at once to get an overview of the program, and then follow it over the next three months—or you can start on a different week, depending on where you are and what your individual goals are. If you get sidetracked, you can always pick up where you left off, or use the chapters to brush up on ways to eat better, become more active, and live a healthier, less stressed, happier life.

The choice is yours. Ready to see how small changes add up to big results? I'll show you.

before you begin the 12-week wellness plan

get the lay of the land

I'm going to help you determine where you are in terms of your current nutrition, activity level, and lifestyle. Are you already eating well but unused to exercise? Do you work out regularly but still feel overwhelmed by stress? Or is your entire lifestyle in need of an overhaul?

You may be tempted to skip this step—I can hear you already, "Come on, come on! I'm ready! Just tell me what to do!" But before you launch into the 12-Week Wellness Plan, take a few minutes to lay the groundwork. You'll have a sense of your biggest obstacles and get a better handle on what specifically you want to improve. And you'll have a solid "before" marker, so when you've completed the plan you can see how far you've come.

To make this easy for you, I've developed a Lifestyle Questionnaire (page 25). After you've taken this 30-question quiz and compiled your scores, you'll immediately have a clearer picture of what areas of your life need improvement—and a realistic idea of what you can accomplish in the next 12 weeks.

the food and exercise journal

The first thing I'm asking you to do is get a notebook—small enough to carry with you everywhere—and start a *Food and Exercise Journal*. This is a place to write down what you're eating and when, how much you exercised, and how you felt afterward, and a way to keep track of the small changes you'll make during the 12-Week Wellness Plan.

You may be resistant to the idea and wonder why you have to *write* everything down. Maybe you're thinking that you'll just skip this step and do the program without the journal.

Let me explain why this journal is so important and helpful. First of all, studies show that people who keep track of how much they eat have an easier time losing and maintaining their weight. Simply writing down what you consume and when makes you more aware of your caloric intake. More than that, maintaining a food and fitness journal becomes a motivational tool in itself. You'll be able to identify your eating and activity patterns, review your progress, and track your improvement in the weeks to come.

Still need convincing? Listen to the story of 40-year-old Jerry, a former client of mine. He came to me in a panic. His older brother had just had a heart attack. Fortunately, his brother had come through okay, but their father had died of heart disease in his late sixties. Jerry feared he was next. He was overweight and knew he had to make some changes in his diet, but he didn't know where to begin.

The first thing I had Jerry do was start a food journal. He wrote down everything he ate and drank, even if it was just a nibble or a sip. After a few days of journal-keeping, one of Jerry's biggest challenges became crystal clear: Jerry was a nibbler. Every time he opened the refrigerator, he'd pop a piece of cheese into his mouth. When he walked by the front desk at his office, he'd grab a handful of candy from the bowl.

When we looked at his food journal together, Jerry was amazed. He couldn't believe how much all the nibbling added up to. When he stopped mindlessly munching all day long, he was on his way to lasting weight loss.

Jerry found the journal an invaluable tool. He had been eating without thinking about it, and keeping the journal helped make him aware of his eating habits. Over time, he found that he could also use the journal to help him stay on track. Keeping the journal sometimes prevented him from overeating, because he shuddered at the thought of writing down three or four doughnuts, or a sleeve of Oreos. He also enjoyed looking back to see how his eating had improved over time.

A few months later, and thirty pounds thinner, Jerry was able to keep track of his eating without keeping a daily journal. He had learned new, healthier eating habits. But even now, he sometimes relies on it as a maintenance tool when he feels he's getting off track and records for a week or two what he eats.

The most important aspect of the journal isn't how big or fancy it looks—it's using it every day. Choose something that's easy to carry that slips into your pocket or purse. That's all there is to it.

the "dear me" letter

Now take a few minutes to write an important letter—to yourself. Write down all the reasons you want to make a positive change in your health. Is it to have more energy? To look and feel better? To be able to see your children grow up and have kids of their own? To live a more fulfilling, happier life? To look better in your jeans? (Hey, that's okay—a little vanity can be a good thing.)

Write what you want to accomplish and why you want to make this positive change. Be as honest as possible—this letter is for your eyes only. After you've written the letter and read it over to yourself, keep it with you. If you feel your motivation flagging, take it out and remind yourself of why you're making this change. Regardless of what your spouse, friends, or children want for you, it's you who has to make the effort.

I believe that to make a change in your lifestyle, you must use your *head*, your *heart*, and your *hands*. Let me explain. You need knowledge about what to do (your head), you need the motivation to make the change (your heart), and you need the skills to enact the change (your hands). Your "Dear Me" letter is really the heart of the program—it reminds you of why you're doing this. When your life gets in the way—when you feel too tired to go for a 20-minute walk or you're tempted to skip your healthy snack in favor of a big chocolate chip cookie—take out the letter and reread it. It can help keep you on track when you're tempted to stray.

asking for—and receiving—support

Another thing that can help keep you on track is the support of the people around you. The changes you make have an impact on your family, friends, and coworkers, and their response to your new behaviors can make a tremendous difference. Your family will be affected when you stop keeping a lot of chips and cookies around the house and begin preparing different kinds of foods. Your coworkers will notice that you are going for walks during your lunch break instead of joining them at the greasy spoon. If the people in your life find your new behaviors threatening, or they don't understand why you are doing things differently, they may be discouraging or try to pressure you to go back to your old ways.

So let everyone know you've decided to take better care of yourself, and tell them you need their help. Ask your family to help choose among the recipes in this book and to keep junk food out of your sight. Invite your coworkers to join you on your walks. Perhaps there is a friend who shares your desire for change and a healthy lifestyle. With the backing of the people in your life, you'll be much more likely to succeed.

Another great way to get support is to ask someone to work through the program with you. Has your neighbor said she'd like to lose some weight? Enlist her, and the two of you can help keep each other on track.

the numbers game

The Lifestyle Questionnaire, food and exercise journal, and the "Dear Me" letter are all valuable tools, but sometimes there is no substitute for hard numbers. If you are "weigh-o-phobic" or tend to obsess over a number on the scale, you can skip this step. But if you're up to the challenge, weigh yourself before you start the program. If you hate the scale, simply measure your chest, waist, and hips with a tape measure—the numbers may surprise (or shock!) you, but remember they're only numbers. Like the Lifestyle Questionnaire, they'll give you a starting point.

If, like many people, you like hard evidence to prove your progress, you'll now have the figures you need. Make a note of them here—you'll compare the end results at the end of the 12 weeks. There is also a space at the end of each chapter to record your weight. Again, if you feel that regular weighing is not for you, feel free to skip this step. However, data from the National Weight Control Registry shows that regular weighing in is one of the habits of people who have successfully lost weight and kept it off.

Date ....   **Chest** (inches) ....

Weight ....   **Waist** (inches) ....

                                                  Hips (inches) ....

lifestyle questionnaire

how healthy are you?

Maybe you need to lose weight, but you're pretty good about balancing the demands of your daily life. Or maybe you already eat healthfully but can't seem to find the motivation to exercise. Taking the Lifestyle Questionnaire will give you insight into how healthy your lifestyle is already—and what areas you can improve upon.

As you answer, be honest with yourself. Don't select the answer that you'd like to say is true; choose the one that best fits your lifestyle now. Regardless of whether you score on the low side—or do better than you thought—you'll have a snapshot of your current habits to compare your progress to in the future.

nutrition check

1. Do you agree with the following statement? "I'm usually aware of what and how much I'm eating."

   a. Yes—I try to pay attention to my food because I enjoy it more.

   b. It depends on how busy I am and whether I'm eating solo or with others.

   c. No—in fact, I often eat at my desk, in the car, or while watching television.

2. How often do you feel "stuffed" or overly full after eating?

   a. Rarely.

   b. Occasionally.

   c. Quite often.

3. How often do you skip meals? (And coffee doesn't count as breakfast.)

   a. Rarely.

   b. Sometimes—it depends on my schedule or if I'm not hungry.

   c. Frequently—I don't eat breakfast, and lunch is often on the run.

4. How may 8-ounce glasses of water do you consume on an average day?

   a. Five glasses or more.

   b. Two to five glasses.

   c. Less than two glasses.

5. How often do you snack on chips or other junk food? (Be honest.)

   a. Rarely—and I pay attention to my portions.

   b. A few times a week.

   c. Frequently—I need my salt or sugar dose every day.

6. What type of protein do you usually consume?

   a. Fish, beans, skinless chicken breast, extra-lean beef, or pork.

   b. Chicken with the skin, or trimmed beef or pork.

   c. Hamburgers, hot dogs, sausages, or marbled steaks.

continues ›››

7. Your diet includes beans, nuts, and soy products:

a. Frequently and often.
b. Occasionally.
c. Rarely.

8. How many servings of fruits and vegetables do you eat? (See Appendix C, page 294 for serving sizes.)

a. Five or more servings a day.
b. Three or four servings a day.
c. Less than two servings a day . . . and that's counting french fries.

9. How many servings of dairy or other high-calcium foods do you consume every day? (See Calcium-Rich Foods on page 278 for serving sizes and examples.)

a. Three or more.
b. One or two.
c. Less than one a day.

10. You incorporate whole grains into your diet:

a. Whenever possible.
b. Occasionally—you ask for whole wheat bread instead of white, for example.
c. Rarely.

fitness check

11. How long can you walk fast without getting out of breath?

a. Easily 30 minutes or more.
b. For 5 to 10 minutes.
c. Less than 5 minutes.

12. Think back to high school. How does your current weight compare with your weight then?

a. It's about the same.
b. It's gone up between 10 and 20 pounds.
c. It's gone up 20 pounds or more.

13. How often do you exercise for at least 20 minutes at a stretch?

a. I exercise three to five days a week, often vigorously.
b. I exercise two or three days a week, but I rarely break a sweat.
c. I don't exercise much at all.

14. How often do you stretch?

a. At least three times a week.
b. Once a week, when I think of it, or when I know it would feel good.
c. Never.

15. How often do you strength-train or lift weights?

a. Two or three times a week.
b. Rarely—I don't want to bulk up.
c. Never.

16. When was the last time you had fun during exercise?

a. Within the last couple of days—I enjoy my usual routine.
b. Recently, playing ball with friends or chasing my kids.
c. I can't remember the last time I had fun exercising; it always feels like a chore to me.

17. When was the last time you tried a new physical activity, whether alone or with someone else?

    a. In the last month.
    b. In the last six months.
    c. I can't remember.

18. Your spouse or friend has suggested a hiking trip this weekend. Your reaction?

    a. Great! It will be a chance to spend some fun time together.
    b. But I have so much to do—I can't afford the time.
    c. No way!

19. How often do you perform some form of sustained physical activity (like walking, gardening, or doing housework) for at least 20 minutes?

    a. Five times a week or more.
    b. Three or four times a week.
    c. Rarely.

20. How satisfied are you with the overall state of your physical body?

    a. Pretty satisfied.
    b. I'd like to lose some weight and/or tone up.
    c. I'd like to lose a lot of weight and completely reshape my body.

wellness check

21. How easy is it for you to relax at the end of the day?

    a. It depends on the day. It is easy on most days.
    b. It's difficult on many days.
    c. It's impossible. I couldn't relax even if I had the time.

22. How often do you eat to comfort yourself or relieve stress?

    a. Rarely.
    b. Sometimes.
    c. Often.

23. How often do you feel like you're living the life you want to?

    a. Frequently.
    b. Occasionally.
    c. Almost never.

24. You'd describe your desk at work or home as:

    a. Fairly organized.
    b. Pretty disorganized, but I know where the important piles are.
    c. A complete mess.

25. Which answer best describes how you use your cell phone or smartphone (whether texting, e-mailing, or making/taking calls)?

    a. I use it for necessary communication and socializing but can easily turn it off when I want to.
    b. I often feel chained to it, but I am comfortable shutting it off for some downtime.
    c. I feel it has taken over my life and can't seem to put it down, even at dinner or on vacation.

continues ›››

26. How would you describe your sleep habits?

    a. I usually feel rested when I wake up.

    b. I could use extra sleep most mornings.

    c. I need a forklift to get out of bed.

27. How often do you feel emotionally out of control?

    a. Rarely, unless I'm under extreme stress.

    b. Occasionally.

    c. Frequently.

28. How often do you take time to do something just for you?

    a. Every day.

    b. Occasionally.

    c. Are you kidding? I have a job and a family—I don't have time just for me!

29. How many close friends would you say you have?

    a. Several.

    b. One, but I can talk to him/her about anything.

    c. I'm not that close to anyone.

30. When you think about the future, how do you feel?

    a. Excited—I have lots to look forward to.

    b. Worried that I'll never catch up on everything I have to do.

    c. I try not to think about the future—it's too overwhelming.

Done? Now take a moment and add up your answers for each of the three sections. Give yourself 5 points for every a, 3 points for every b, and 1 point for every c answer, and write down your score:

Nutrition Score: .... (out of a possible 50)

Fitness Score: .... (out of a possible 50)

Wellness Score: .... (out of a possible 50)

DATE
....

Total Score: .... (out of a possible 150)

Take a look at your score, and consider the areas of your life that you'd like to improve. Once you have completed the 12-Week Wellness Plan, you will retake the test and have measurable proof of your progress toward a healthy life. Now, if you've written your "Dear Me" letter and have your designated notebook, you're ready to embark on the plan! Let's begin. . . .

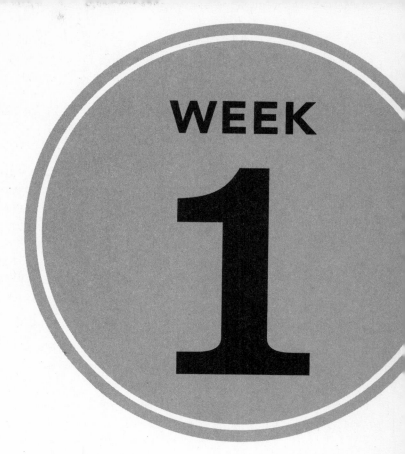

WEEK 1

this week's changes

1. Shop and get comfortable with a healthy pantry.

2. Start walking for 20 minutes, three times a week.

3. Practice the Five-Minute Breathing Exercise daily.

this week's recipes

Rush-Hour Dinners in 15 Minutes or Less

- Cuban-Style Black Beans
- Lemon Pepper Chicken
- Linguini with Shrimp
- Honey Mustard Salmon

This week's Eating Well change starts in the kitchen, where you will revamp your pantry, filling it with the most healthful ingredients. With your new, well-stocked kitchen and these quick, easy recipes, you will see how doable it can be to have healthy, satisfying meals even on the busiest weekdays.

cuban-style black beans

SERVES 6 *These flavorful beans can be served as a side, with rotisserie chicken, say, and they also make a hearty main dish when piled over rice. A salad of sliced tomato, avocado, and red onion dressed with olive oil and lime juice is a perfect accompaniment.*

2 (15.5-ounce) cans of black beans, preferably low-sodium
1 tablespoon olive oil
1 medium onion, diced (about 1 cup)
1 green bell pepper, diced (about 1 cup)
2 garlic cloves, minced
¼ teaspoon dried oregano
1 teaspoon cumin
3 tablespoons cider vinegar
¼ cup dry sherry or white wine
Salt and freshly ground black pepper to taste

1. Drain the beans in a colander and rinse gently under cold water.

2. Heat the oil in a medium saucepan over a medium flame, add the onion, and cook for 3 minutes. Add the pepper and cook 3 minutes more, stirring occasionally. Add the garlic and cook for 1 minute. Stir in the beans, oregano, cumin, vinegar, sherry or wine, and ½ cup of water. Simmer on low for 5 minutes. Season with salt and pepper before serving.

Calories 160; Fat 2.5 g (Sat 0 g, Mono 1.7 g, Poly 0.3 g); Protein 8 g; Carb 25 g; Fiber 8 g; Chol 0 mg; Sodium 140 mg

lemon pepper chicken

SERVES 4 *Mark Bittman, cookbook author and New York Times columnist, showed me a version of this simple and delicious recipe when he was a guest on my very first TV show, Living Better. It has been a rush-hour staple in my house ever since.*

- **1 to 1½ pounds boneless chicken breast, pounded to a uniform ½-inch thickness**
- **½ teaspoon coarse salt**
- **1 teaspoon freshly ground black pepper**
- **2 teaspoons olive oil**
- **¼ cup freshly squeezed lemon juice**

1. Pat the chicken breasts dry and season both sides with the salt and pepper.

2. Heat the olive oil in a large nonstick skillet over a medium-high flame. Place the chicken in the pan and cook for 6 to 8 minutes, turning once. Turn off the heat and pour the lemon juice over the chicken. Serve.

Calories 160; Fat 1.8 g (Sat .5 g, Mono .4 g, Poly .4 g); Protein 32.8 g; Carb 1.3 g; Fiber 1 g; Chol 82 mg; Sodium 333 mg

linguini with shrimp

SERVES 4 *I always have frozen shrimp on hand to make easy, elegant meals practically instantly. This lemony pasta dish sprinkled with fresh parsley is one of my family's favorites. Serve with a simple green salad, or sliced tomatoes drizzled with olive oil, for a delightful, express dinner.*

¾ pound whole-grain linguini
2 tablespoons olive oil
2 garlic cloves, minced
1 pound large shrimp, peeled and deveined
⅓ cup freshly squeezed lemon juice
½ cup white wine
1 cup chopped fresh, flat-leaf parsley
¼ teaspoon salt, plus more to taste
Freshly ground black pepper to taste

1. Bring a large pot of water to a boil. Add the linguini and cook according to the directions on the box. Drain, reserving 1 cup of the cooking water.

2. Meanwhile, heat the olive oil in a large skillet over a medium-high flame. Add the garlic and sauté for 1 minute. Add the shrimp and cook for 3 to 4 minutes, until the shrimp turn pink. Remove the shrimp from the pan and set aside. Add the lemon juice, white wine, and the reserved cup of pasta water to the skillet. Let simmer until the liquid is reduced by about half. Return the shrimp to the pan and stir in the parsley.

3. Add the drained linguini to the shrimp mixture, tossing to combine. Season with salt and pepper.

Calories 510; Fat 10g (Sat 1.5 g, Mono 5.4 g, Poly 2.0 g); Protein 36 g; Carb 69 g; Fiber 11 g; Chol 170 mg; Sodium 330 mg

honey mustard salmon

SERVES 4 *Whenever someone tells me they don't have time to cook, I give them this recipe to prove them wrong. Just a few simple ingredients and 10 to 15 minutes are all it takes to bring a flavorful, satisfying and healthy entrée to the table. While the salmon is cooking, steam some broccoli to serve alongside.*

Cooking spray
¼ cup Dijon mustard, preferably whole-grain
2 tablespoons honey
Four 6-ounce salmon fillets

1. Preheat the oven to 350°F. Spray a baking sheet with cooking spray. In a small bowl, mix together the mustard and honey to combine.

2. Place the salmon fillets onto the baking sheet and spoon the honey mustard mixture generously over each fillet. Put the fillets in the oven and cook for 10 minutes per inch thickness or until desired doneness, and serve.

Calories 290; Fat 11 g (Sat 1.7 g, Mono 3.6 g, Poly 4.3 g); Protein 34 g; Carb 12 g; Fiber 0 g; Chol 95 mg; Sodium 440 mg

Welcome to Week 1! You may not realize it, but although you are just beginning, you've done a lot already. By picking up this book, buying it, actually *reading* it, and getting to this point, you've moved from just thinking about changing your life to taking real action. Now let's keep the momentum going and dive into this week's changes.

 # EATING WELL

a healthy pantry

The first step toward eating well is having nutritious food at your fingertips. You can have the best intentions in the world, but if you have nothing good in your refrigerator, that's most likely what you'll wind up eating—nothing good. Sure, you can manage to eat right by relying on restaurants and takeout (see Eight Tips for Dining Out, page 38), but it's tough to do that every day. Studies show that people who eat out often have a much higher sodium and calorie intake than those who prepare more meals at home. And it makes sense. When you cook your own meals, you have the ultimate control over what you are eating. When you have healthy food on hand, you never have to worry about what you're going to eat next, and you're less likely to succumb to impulsive snacking and overeating. In short, having a stocked pantry takes the stress out of eating well and helps you stay on track.

You may be thinking you don't have time to shop for and prepare healthy meals. But you do—because I am going to help you make the process easy and efficient. Once you invest a little time in stocking your pantry, you'll have everything you need to whip up a healthy meal faster than you can order a pizza. In this book I've given you 65 easy, enticing recipes. You'll also have plenty of "eat-on-the-run" foods that you can grab as you head out the door. And you'll save money by forgoing all those restaurant and takeout meals.

First, look in your fridge, freezer, and cupboard, and take inventory of what you have. Toss any frozen "mystery meat" and canned foods that have been in your home since you moved in—you know, the things like canned pumpkin that you never got around to using for Thanksgiving six years ago.

healthy shopping list

fresh vegetables and herbs

- Asparagus
- Avocado
- Basil
- Bell peppers
- Broccoli
- Cabbage
- Carrots
- Cauliflower
- Celery
- Cilantro
- Collard greens
- Corn
- Cucumbers
- Eggplant
- Garlic
- Ginger
- Green beans
- Kale
- Leeks
- Lettuce
- Mint
- Mushrooms
- Onions
- Parsley
- Potatoes
- Radishes
- Rosemary
- Scallions
- Spinach
- Sweet potatoes
- Swiss chard
- Thyme
- Tomatoes
- Winter squash
- Zucchini
- Other ....

fruits and juices

- Apple cider
- Apples
- Apricots, dried or fresh
- Bananas
- Blackberries
- Blueberries
- Cantaloupe
- Cherries, dried or fresh
- Cranberries, dried or fresh
- Figs, dried or fresh
- Grapefruit
- Grapefruit juice
- Grapes
- Honeydew
- Kiwifruit
- Lemons
- Limes
- Nectarines
- Orange juice
- Oranges
- Peaches
- Pears
- Pineapple
- Plums
- Raisins
- Raspberries
- Strawberries
- Tangerines
- Watermelon
- Other ....

beans, nuts, and seeds

- Almond butter
- Almonds
- Dried beans
- Lentils
- Peanut butter
- Pecans
- Pine nuts
- Pistachios
- Sesame seeds
- Split peas
- Walnuts
- Other ....

spices and dried herbs

- Allspice
- Basil
- Bay leaves
- Black pepper
- Cayenne pepper
- Chili powder
- Chipotle chili powder
- Cinnamon, ground
- Coriander, ground
- Cumin, ground
- Curry powder
- Garlic powder
- Ginger, ground
- Oregano
- Paprika
- Red pepper, crushed
- Rosemary
- Sage
- Salt
- Tarragon
- Thyme
- Turmeric
- Vanilla extract, pure
- Other ....

continues ›››

dairy and soy

- 1% or nonfat milk
- Feta cheese
- Low-fat buttermilk
- Low-fat cottage cheese
- Low-fat or nonfat yogurt, regular and Greek-style
- Parmesan cheese
- Part-skim mozzarella
- Part-skim ricotta
- Sharp Cheddar
- Soy milk
- Tofu
- Other ....

oils and condiments

- All-fruit preserves
- Balsamic vinegar
- Brown sugar, light and dark
- Canola mayonnaise
- Canola oil
- Cider vinegar
- Cooking spray
- Grapeseed oil
- Honey
- Ketchup
- Molasses
- Mustard
- Natural cocoa powder
- Olive oil
- Olives
- Peanut oil
- Pure maple syrup
- Red wine
- Red wine vinegar
- Sesame oil
- Sherry or wine for cooking
- Soy sauce, low-sodium
- Tea: green, black, herbal
- Walnut oil
- White wine
- White wine vinegar
- Worcestershire sauce
- Other ....

grains and baking Items

- All-purpose flour
- Baked tortilla chips
- Baking powder
- Baking soda
- Brown rice
- Brown rice flour
- Bulgur
- Corn tortillas
- Cornmeal
- Cornstarch
- Flax, ground
- Oatmeal
- Quinoa
- Whole-grain cold cereal
- Whole-grain crackers
- Whole-grain dinner rolls
- Whole-grain pasta
- Whole wheat bread
- Whole wheat couscous
- Whole wheat flour
- Whole wheat pastry flour
- Whole wheat pita
- Wild rice
- Other ....

fresh meats, poultry, and fish

- Beef, extra-lean
- Chicken breast, skinless
- Eggs
- Fish
- Ground turkey, lean
- Ham, extra-lean
- Pork tenderloin, loin
- Poultry sausage
- Scallops
- Shrimp
- Turkey breast, skinless
- Venison
- Other ....

canned/jarred (low-sodium whenever possible)

- Applesauce (no sugar added)
- Beans, black
- Beans, white
- Beef broth
- Chicken broth
- Garbanzo beans
- Kidney beans
- Pesto sauce
- Pineapple (in juice)
- Salmon
- Sardines
- Tomato juice
- Tomato paste
- Tomato sauce
- Tomatoes, crushed
- Tomatoes, diced
- Tuna in water
- Other ....

frozen

- Broccoli
- Corn
- Edamame
- Peas
- Spinach
- Stir-fry medley
- Vegetable medley
- Veggie burgers
- Whole-grain waffles
- Winter squash
- Other ....

storage guidelines

FOOD	STORAGE FOR PEAK QUALITY
canned foods	
High-acid foods (tomatoes, pineapple)	12–18 months
Low-acid foods (most vegetables, meats, poultry, fish)	2–5 years
frozen foods	
Cooked leftovers	2–6 months
Fish, uncooked	3–6 months
Frozen dinners and entrées	3–4 months
Ground meat and poultry, stew meat, uncooked	3–4 months
Poultry, uncooked	9–12 months
Sausage, hot dogs, lunch meat	1–2 months
Steaks, roasts, and chops, uncooked	4–12 months
packaged/dried foods	
Cereal, opened	2–3 months
Cereal, unopened	6–12 months
Dried beans	1 year
Pasta, rice (in airtight container)	1 year
Peanut butter, unopened	6–9 months

eight tips for dining out

Eating out? Join the club—most of us eat about one in three meals away from home, and that can be bad news for your waistline. Restaurant meals tend to be higher in calories and sodium than eating at home, for several reasons. First, the portions are often oversize—studies reveal that the average restaurant portion is often two to three times a "normal" serving. Second, restaurants tend to be pretty heavy-handed with fat, salt, and sugar. You can still eat out and eat healthy, but it takes a little thought, and sometimes some extra planning.

Give these tips a try:

1. **Choose wisely.** Yes, you can order healthfully in just about any restaurant, but make it easier by choosing a place that's known for serving healthfully prepared food. Restaurants specializing in seafood or produce that is local or seasonal are usually a good bet.

2. **Plan ahead.** If you haven't eaten at your restaurant choice before, check out its website. Most restaurants now include their menus online; some include calorie and nutrient info, as well. Decide what to order before you get there so that you are less likely to make an impulsive decision at the table.

3. **Look for the magic words:** *steamed, poached, broiled, roasted, grilled,* and *baked.* These are the most healthful preparations of foods. Avoid dishes with descriptions like *fried, crispy, battered, creamy/creamed, cheesy, dipped,* or *deep-fried.* Check the menu; many chain restaurants now indicate healthy choices with a symbol.

4. **Be assertive.** Not sure how a dish is prepared? Ask your server. And don't be afraid to make special requests. You can ask that sauces and dressings be served on the side, that food be broiled or steamed without butter, or that a dish be made without cheese, for example. Most restaurants are happy to accommodate their guests.

5. Keep portions human-size. You know now that "portion" is more likely to be two or three actual servings. (See Appendix C, Serving Sizes.) Don't feel compelled to clean your plate; try these ways to keep portions sensible:

- Order two appetizers, or an appetizer and a salad, instead of an appetizer and an entrée.

- Order an entrée to split in half—either to share with a dining partner or to take home for another meal.

6. Pass the bread basket. It's practically impossible to resist a basket of chips or warm bread put right in front of you at a restaurant while you're hungry. Ask your server not to put it out at all or at least wait until the meal arrives so that you are less likely to fill up on it.

7. Start with soup or salad. Studies show that if you start a meal with a healthy soup or salad, you wind up eating fewer calories throughout the meal. So order a light appetizer like a garden salad, vegetable soup, consommé, or grilled vegetables to start your meal, and you'll be ahead of the game.

8. Desert dessert. Are you in the habit of having dessert after every meal? Break it and do the unthinkable: say "no thanks" to dessert. If that's too drastic, opt for sorbet, fresh fruit, or a mini-dessert (a small portion) that many restaurants now offer.

Then, using the Healthy Shopping List (page 35) as a guide, make note of what you need and head out to the store. Keep in mind that although there are a wealth of delicious, good-for-you grocery items to explore that are not on the Healthy Shopping List, as the list is meant to be a starting point, it is still quite extensive—it contains all the ingredients you'll need to make any recipe in this book. So don't feel like you must buy everything on the list! You may want to look at the recipes peppered throughout the book and purchase the ingredients for the ones you want to try first. Ultimately, you'll pick and choose what you like (and what your family likes) and in appropriate amounts for you and your family.

Approach this initial shopping as the time to stock up on nonperishables. Buying bulk quantities of rice; cereals; and canned, frozen, and dried foods will free you to do just a light weekly shopping for the next month or so, and will save you money.

After your initial "stock-up" shopping trip, pick a convenient day and time to do your weekly shopping hereafter, and stick to it. If your schedule is flexible, you might ask the supermarket manager when the store receives fresh produce, and plan to shop on one of those days—you'll have a nicer selection to choose from. I recommend that each week you buy ingredients for salad (prewashed greens are a real time saver), four or five other fresh vegetables, and four or five different fresh fruits, depending on what looks most appealing and what's in season. That will get you in the habit of eating more fruits and vegetables and introduce you to new ones.

Another tip: if you eat on the go a lot, buy individual servings of foods like yogurt, cottage cheese, tuna, and applesauce so that you'll have them handy. Having a stash of nuts and "portable" fruit like bananas, apples, and grapes also makes it easy to grab a few healthy snacks on your way out the door.

The foods on this shopping list may look familiar from my Usually/Sometimes/Rarely food lists on pages 14–16. You'll notice that the Healthy Shopping List contains nearly all the Usually foods and a few Sometimes foods. So, while the only change you need to make this week is to establish a healthy pantry, I have an ulterior motive—to get you to start eating those wonderful foods I recommend for an ideal diet.

Take a look in your cupboard again. How many of the foods there are on the Rarely list? If your house is loaded with Rarely items and you feel they will distract you from your new, healthier foods, consider giving away those foods to a neighbor or throwing them out. You don't have to get rid of them if you don't want to, but at least store them out of sight so that your new and improved pantry takes center stage.

the power of the pen: the food journal

Once you've gotten your pantry whipped into shape, begin to record in your journal everything you eat and drink. As I explained on page 21, this is an amazingly effective, eye-opening exercise for most people. Many of us are accustomed to eating unconsciously, munching on whatever comes our way or tempts us at the moment. When it comes down to it, most of us have only a vague idea of how much we consume and our eating patterns. Writing down what you eat brings consciousness to your eating. It forces you to be aware of what and how much you eat and allows you to look back and see how you are doing.

Your journal should look something like this: Write down when you ate, what foods you had, the amounts (estimates are fine), and, if you like, how you felt afterward. I strongly recommend that you make entries throughout the day, as you eat, instead of filling it in each night, trying to remember what you had and when (you'll forget stuff, believe me!). If you are dining out and don't want to write in your journal at the table, you can take a quick photo of your plate of food, or jot the meal down in the car right afterward. Keeping the journal may seem like a nuisance at first, but stick to it—it will help you stay conscious of your eating and make you more aware of your usual habits.

	Monday, March 8		
time	food or beverage consumed	amount	notes
7:30	oatmeal	1 cup	felt satisfied
	1% milk	1 cup	
	raisins	2 tablespoons	

action

The first part of your action plan this week is to go shopping to revamp your pantry. The second component is simply keeping your food journal—writing down what you eat, when you eat, and how much. That's all there is to it.

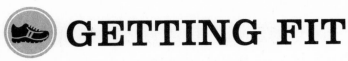

GETTING FIT

the walking plan

Are you ready for the fitness part of the plan? If you're like many people, you're brimming with enthusiasm and good intentions. You're ready to get in shape, and you want results *fast*—like yesterday.

Slow down just a bit. When many people start exercising, they jump in head-first. But overdoing it can lead to sore muscles, a sense of being overwhelmed, or even injury. My plan will let you embark on your fitness plan at a safe, moderate pace that will prevent those aches and pains you may associate with exercise.

The object of this week is simple—to get you moving on a regular basis.

WHY WALK? It's so basic that we do it every day without thinking about it, but believe it or not, *walking* is the easiest way to get and stay fit. Even if you've never worked out before, you'll find it an efficient, effective method of exercise. And if you're an experienced exerciser, a regular walking routine may be easier to maintain than a more complicated program—you can walk practically anywhere with a pair of comfortable shoes as the only necessary equipment.

While you could use any form of aerobic exercise for the fitness component of my 12-Week Wellness Plan, I chose walking for Week 1 because of its universality. If you like, though, feel free to substitute another aerobic activity, such as biking, and follow the same workout program. The key is to enjoy what you're doing. So, if walking is not for you, or not ideal because of where you live or work, then choose something you do like—you'll find it easier to stick with. Or mix it up by walking two days a week and biking one day, if that makes it more fun for you.

Sometimes people find it hard to believe that simply walking can make such a big difference in the way they feel. But take Emma, a 38-year-old secretary at a law school. Though Emma was committed to exercising regularly, with three school-age boys at home and a stressful job, the reality was that she found it nearly impossible to find the time to work out. She belonged to a local gym, but she was lucky to get there once a week. On top of that, the stress from work was taking a toll on her. She'd often find herself munching on the doughnuts and cookies that were always around the office to take the edge off during the day. Then at night, she'd have trouble unwinding and falling asleep.

Eventually Emma gave up the idea of going to the gym and started walking during her lunch hour. Since she could eat lunch at her desk afterward, she was able to keep to a fairly regular walking schedule. And when she organized a lunch-time walking group with three of her coworkers, her fitness regimen really took off.

Five years later, Emma is 10 pounds lighter, and what's important is that she has kept the weight off. She's better able to cope with the demands of her job. She walks with her group every day, Monday through Friday—indoors during the snowy Michigan winter and outdoors when the weather is good. "You won't cop out when someone else is depending on you," says Emma. "We encourage each other, push each other to walk a little faster, and the time goes faster." She says she doesn't even think about whether or not she is going to walk that day. It's automatic.

Besides giving her more energy and relieving stress, Emma says her walking eliminates her urge to eat junk food at work, because she wants to hang on to the healthy feeling she gets from exercising regularly. She also finds it much easier to sleep at night. Emma believes her walking group has really made her life better, and she encourages people to find at least one person to walk with. "It makes it more regular, and more fun," she says.

FINDING THE TIME Emma faced one of the biggest reasons for not exercising—lack of time. That's one reason I'm having you start with a small time commit-ment—20 minutes, three times a week. But if you're wondering just when you're going to carve out even that small sliver of time, take a close look at your daily schedule. Can you walk first thing in the morning before your kids get up? During your lunch hour at work? While your daughter has piano lessons? Or perhaps there's a weekly errand you do where you can walk instead of drive. Twenty minutes isn't a lot of time, and if you need to break it up into smaller chunks (say, two 10-minute sessions), that's fine, too.

One of the easiest ways to commit to an exercise program is to write it down in your calendar or date book, the way you would any other appointment. After all, it's an appointment with yourself—and an investment in your overall health and fitness. At the beginning of the week, figure out when you'll put in your three sessions. Will you walk at lunch Monday, Wednesday, and Friday? Or get up early Tuesday and Thursday, and then walk around the soccer field during your son's game Saturday morning? Write down when you'll exercise and stick to it.

STAYING MOTIVATED Some people find that the best way for them to keep to a regular regimen is to keep to the same route, covering the same blocks if they walk in town, or the same lanes or back roads if they walk in the suburbs or country. People who thrive on routine also try to find a regular time of day that is convenient, such as first thing in the morning or just before dinner, which helps them keep to a regular schedule. Very quickly, such regularity can allow you to "zone out," to think about other things as you walk, or to almost "meditate" as you exercise.

However, other people find such regularity and sameness incredibly boring. If this sounds like you, consider adding a number of variations to your three-times-a-week walks. The easiest way to avoid boredom as you walk is simply to take different routes. For example, walk through a park one day, along the river the next, through a new neighborhood on the third day.

Many people enjoy walking in malls, which allows them to window-shop as they walk and offers protection from the elements, since most malls are covered. Some schools and colleges open their gym facilities to people in the neighborhood; walking on an indoor track at your local health club or YMCA is another option. Finally, if you have extra time on a weekend, drive to a park or other beautiful setting for a change of scenery.

If you're a new mom, you might want to combine your walking regimen with that of another new mom. You may even want to bring along the babies. If you have older children, walking with them gives you an opportunity to catch up with them. And if you belong to a senior center or YMCA, post a sign seeking a fellow walker. Or encourage your spouse or partner to join you. Walking with a partner makes it all more fun, and it tends to help you avoid procrastinating, keep up a

Connect with Other Walkers

Once you're in a good walking groove, you will likely look forward to your walks. If you need a little extra push, though, you'll find a slew of websites where you can track your progress, connect with other walkers, and stay motivated. Here are three of my favorites:

- **www.thewalkingsite.com/index.html**
  This site includes message boards, motivation tips, and a list of local clubs you can join.

- **www.the-fitness-walking-guide.com/walking-log.html**
  Want another way to track your progress? Download the walking log from this site.

- **www.realage.com/shape-up-slim-down/walking
  5-ways-to-make-walking-a-habit**
  Register with the site and you can sign up for the online walking tracker; it's a great tool for tracking your walks over months or even years.

vigorous pace, and stay on course with your regimen. Having a partner to walk with also allows you to maintain—and even stimulate—your social life as you exercise.

If you have a dog, you can work your dog-walking duties into your walking regimen. Your pet will enjoy the exercise as much as you do and benefit from it, as well. Also, think about teaming up with another dog-owning neighbor or friend.

Walking on a treadmill is one of the most effective ways to establish and maintain a walking routine, if that is your preference. Treadmills are the most popular machines at health clubs; they allow you to precisely monitor your pace, time, distance covered, and calories burned. On a treadmill, you can walk at any time of day or night, no matter what the weather is. Virtually all gyms have treadmills, or you can buy one and use it in the privacy of your home. (Having your own treadmill can make it easier to fit exercise into your schedule, but high-quality, safe treadmills run at least a thousand dollars. So hold off on purchasing one until you're sure it's worth the investment.)

THE PRACTICALITY OF A PEDOMETER One of the best—and least expensive—motivational techniques I know of is the pedometer, a small device that measures the number of steps you take and can be clipped onto your belt or waistband. At a cost of less than $15, it's an inexpensive tool to help you track how much you're moving.

You may have heard the recommendation that people should take 10,000 steps a day to maintain good health, and a pedometer lets you see how close to that goal you're getting as you progress with the 12-week plan, while giving you an incentive to move more, as well. It's a fun way to track your walks and the rest of your daily physical activities, and you may be surprised by how much—or how little—you've been moving. Studies show that people who wear pedometers wind up walking significantly more than those who do not. Taking 10,000 steps is the equivalent of walking about five miles for most people, and that amount of activity is close to what the Centers for Disease Control (CDC) recommend to improve and maintain good health.

You can pick up a pedometer at any sporting goods store or online. Some higher-tech models (about $30) include functions that tell you how far you've traveled and how many calories you've burned, but all you need is a simple step counter. (Before you buy one, though, see Shopping for a Monitor, page 69. Many of the high-tech heart monitors include pedometers.)

Hook the pedometer on your waistband, and center it at the midline of your right or left thigh (where the crease in your pants would be.) Reset it to zero at the beginning of the day or walk, and you'll have a simple way of tracking your activity. If you think you're already pretty active, you may be surprised at how few steps you actually take during the day. On the other hand, you may find that it's easier than you think to add a few hundred steps here and there. One of the reasons step counting is such a useful tool is that it doesn't measure just the steps you take during set-aside workout time, it also adds up all the small things you do throughout the day, like taking the stairs instead of the elevator.

Though you needn't have a pedometer to do the 12-Week Wellness Plan, I've found that those who use them find them extremely motivating. Why not give it a try? (Or up the ante by having a step contest with a friend who wants to become more active. Sometimes friendly competition can keep you moving!)

KEEPING COOL IN HOT WEATHER These five tips will help you stay cool in hot weather. Keep in mind, though, that if the temperature or humidity (or both) is high, you may want to walk in an air-conditioned gym or mall.

1. **Walk during the coolest hours of the day.** Early in the morning is usually best in most locales, but if you live near a beach or lake, breezes off the water may cool the air in late afternoon. Avoid walking at midday, when temperatures usually peak.

2. **Avoid direct sunlight.** Walk on the shady side of the street or along tree-lined hiking paths. If shade isn't an option, that's an especially good argument for walking early in the morning or during early-evening hours, when it's cooler outside.

3. **Cover yourself.** Wear a baseball cap, tennis visor, or hat to shade your face. Wear sunscreen to protect your skin, along with sunglasses and light-colored, lightweight clothing.

4. **Drink lots of water.** Before you start your walk, down a large glass of water. If you're going to walk more than 30 minutes, carry a water bottle or stop for another drink during your walk. When you finish, drink another glass of water or two (at least a pint) to keep your body hydrated. Even if you don't notice yourself sweating, you *are* losing moisture; you don't need a soaked shirt to get dehydrated.

5. **Beware of heat sickness.** If you feel dizzy, nauseated, short of breath, chilly, or otherwise unwell, stop immediately, sit down, and drink some water. Don't be afraid to ask someone for assistance or to help you get home. If you suffer from heart disease, diabetes, or any other medical condition, check with your doctor before walking in hot weather.

KEEPING WARM IN COLD WEATHER If you don't like to exercise in the heat, cooler weather can be a blessing. Many people find it invigorating to walk outdoors, even when it is snowing. The key to staying comfortable is dressing in layers and peeling them off as you warm up during your walk.

1. **Start with the bottom layer.** Choose underwear made from fabrics like polypropylene, Coolmax, Thinsulate, or silk, which draws sweat away from your skin. Look for "moisture-wicking" or "wicking fabric" on the label, and avoid cotton undergarments, which can get sweaty, heavy, and uncomfortable.

2. **Add layers.** Include an insulating layer, such as fleece, pile, or down; add another layer if weather dictates; and finish with a comfortable water-resistant jacket. If the temperature permits, tights may be sufficient; if it's very cold, wear tights or long underwear under water-resistant pants or sweatpants.

3. **Use headgear and accessories.** In cold weather, wear a warm hat or ear band to protect your ears; a scarf will keep your neck warm. Slip on gloves or mittens—in particularly cold weather, gloves worn inside a pair of mittens will keep your fingers toasty. Waterproof walking shoes or hiking boots with heavy socks, made of fabric that will wick perspiration, will keep your feet warm. You may also want to take along lip balm, sunscreen, sunglasses, and a bottle of water—even in the cold, you can still get sunburned or dehydrated.

4. **Watch your step.** If the temperature is or has been below freezing, take extra care with your footing. Even after the day warms up, there may be icy or slick patches. If you walk regularly outdoors in cold weather, check out Yaktrax, ice grippers that fit over your shoes to give added traction and stability.

5. **Be smart.** There's cold—and then there's *cold*. Windchill takes into account the outdoor temperature and wind speed, and the lower the windchill, the more dangerous it is to exercise outdoors. You'll find a windchill chart at www.NWS.noaa.gov/om/windchill.

READY, SET, WALK! At the beginning of your walk, start off slowly. Your muscles and ligaments aren't warmed up yet, especially if you walk early in the morning. After about three to five minutes, you can speed up so that you're walking at a comfortable pace. Your mission isn't to overexert yourself, but instead to get your body used to continuous exercise for 20 minutes. Slow your pace for the last several minutes of your walk—this is the cooldown, and it's important because it allows your heart rate to slow down gradually. When you finish, drink at least 8 ounces of water to replenish your fluids.

This first week, you'll walk three times. This is frequent enough so that exercise will begin to be a habit. At the same time, it gives your body (which may be unused to working out) a chance to adapt while minimizing soreness.

WALK RIGHT, WALK TALL You've been doing it since you were a baby, and chances are you probably don't think about the way you walk. But when you're walking for exercise, form becomes more important. When you walk, your head should be up, your chest lifted, and your legs centered under your hips. Your steps should be comfortable, and your arms should swing naturally as you stride along. You should be walking heel, toe, heel, toe—in other words, your heel should strike the ground first, then you roll onto the ball of your foot, and push off with each step.

If you tend to slump when you stand or walk, imagine a string attached to the crown of your head, pulling your body into alignment. Even hunching over a little will make you more prone to injury over the long haul. Proper form helps prevent this. When you walk, occasionally check your form. Your body shouldn't be ramrod straight, but you should maintain good posture. Also, take normal-size comfortable steps; overstriding increases your risk of soreness and injury.

THE WALKER'S CLOSET Be sure you have a good pair of walking shoes. They're designed to support your feet and minimize jarring, and they're well worth the investment. Look for shoes that fit comfortably, leaving a half inch or so in the toe box between the tips of your toes and the end of the shoe itself. They shouldn't pinch your heels nor be so loose that your foot moves freely as you step. If you have high or low arches, you'll want to select a shoe designed for your type of foot.

Your best option is to buy a new pair of shoes at a specialty shoe shop or a fitness store. You may spend a little more than grabbing a pair at your local superstore, but you're also more likely to get a pair of shoes that fit your type of foot. The salesperson may want to look at your feet and the wear patterns of the shoes you're wearing to determine what type of shoe will be best for you. You may be asked how often you walk, on what surfaces, and what distances.

Comfortable socks help support and cushion your feet while you walk. You can walk in any type of socks, but if you tend to get blisters, you may want to try synthetic fabrics over cotton. Socks with CoolMax, Supplex, or other synthetic blends are designed to draw sweat away from your skin, so your feet feel drier and more comfortable. Thin socks may also reduce your chance of blisters—thick socks can bunch up and rub while you're walking.

You can walk in just about any type of clothing, but you don't want to restrict your movement. You may be most comfortable in shorts, sweats, or tights on the bottom and a T-shirt or sweatshirt on top. In cooler weather, dress in layers and a hat and gloves; then you can remove them as you warm up.

To Tune In or Not?

Listening to music while you exercise is a great way to stay motivated—in fact, studies show that people can work out longer and at a higher level when they're "tuned in." Music can be an enjoyable distraction, whether you're strolling at an easy pace or want something to help you pump up your intensity.

If you're planning to exercise to music, consider the tempo of your tunes; higher-tempo music tends to make you exercise more intensely, while slower-tempo music may cause you to slow down without realizing it. If you need a more restorative, easy-paced workout, however, relaxing music can help keep you from overdoing it. And though it seems obvious, choose music you like! Studies show that while music you like makes workouts seem easier, music you don't care for actually makes them seem more challenging.

Smartphones and MP3 players make it easier than ever to have music wherever you go. Some models, like the iPod shuffle, are just larger than a quarter; so you can easily clip them on your waistband. Load up your player with motivating tunes and you'll find that your workout speeds by. (Not a fan of working out to music? If you'd rather listen to an audiobook, check out www.audible.com for thousands of selections to choose from.) Or maybe your walks are your chance to catch up on your favorite weekly podcasts.

A word of caution, though—if you wear earphones or a headset, keep the volume low enough so that you can hear what's happening around you. This will help prevent hearing damage. Also, while it's great to lose yourself in your music, don't do this while walking in high-traffic or crowded areas where you need to pay attention to bikers, rollerbladers, or vehicles.

In addition to your walking clothing, you may want to invest in some safety and reflective gear. If you walk early in the morning or at the end of the day, reflective gear can save your life. You can find hats, gloves, vests, and other articles of clothing that have reflective surfaces as well as flashing lights and other attention-getting equipment that you can strap on your arm or your waistband. Wearing light-colored clothing, especially at dawn and dusk, makes you more visible to drivers, bicyclists, and others.

Want a place to stash your car keys, cell phone, a small towel, and a bottle of

staying safe and walking smart

If you walk indoors, you may be less concerned with safety. But if you're walking outside, a few tips will help keep you healthy and safe. While anyone can be attacked while walking, women are particularly vulnerable, so take precautions:

1. **Walk defensively.** When you're outside, pay attention to your environment and who's around you. Walk with your head up and look at people as they approach you. Don't walk alone in isolated areas.

2. **Look for cars.** The average driver is not looking for you—you're much smaller than another vehicle. Stay off the roads whenever possible, and choose routes away from heavily trafficked areas. As a child you were taught to look both ways before crossing the street, so make sure you do, even at stop signs—many drivers don't bother to stop completely and may not see you. If you must walk in the street, walk on the left side, facing traffic, as far over on the shoulder as you can get. You're much safer facing traffic than walking with it, besides it's the law to do so.

3. **Walk in well-traveled and well-lit places whenever possible—there's safety in numbers.** Know where the nearest house or pay phone is, or carry a cell phone with you in case of an emergency. If you must walk alone after dark, stick close to your home or walk in a place that's relatively busy and well-lit. (For example, a park near my home has baseball and soccer fields that are lighted during summer nights, and many people stroll around the fields after dark.)

4. **Don't carry valuables.** Lock your purse or your wallet in your car, or leave it at home. Don't carry loads of cash or wear expensive jewelry—you'll make yourself a target.

5. **Let someone know.** Even if it is just sending a quick text, tell someone that you are heading out for a walk and how long you expect to be gone. If you're walking in a new locale or park, take a map to keep in your pocket.

water? Grab a carrier or fanny pack, strap it along your waist, and you're ready to go. Make sure that whatever you choose is comfortable and doesn't chafe or irritate your skin; it should fit snugly enough that it doesn't bounce a lot but not so close that it feels tight. You may also want to carry an inexpensive plastic water bottle with a snap-off or squirt cap to help you stay hydrated; some come with straps to make them easier to carry in your hand, while many will fit into a waist carrier designed to hold them.

If your regimen involves walking outside, you'll want to take the season—and the weather—into account. I encourage people to walk outside whenever possible, where you can feel the sun on your face, smell fresh air, hear the sounds of birds, and enjoy your surroundings in a way that isn't possible indoors. Simply being outside can lift your spirits—research shows that people who walk outside feel happier and report a more elevated mood than people who walk the same distance indoors.

FOR WOMEN ONLY You may want to consider one final addition to your walker's wardrobe: a decent sports bra. While walking is a lower-impact activity than jogging, unless you're small-breasted, an athletic bra will help make your walks more enjoyable. (You don't want to worry about bouncing around all over the place, and it's uncomfortable as well!)

There are two basic types of sports bras: compression bras and encapsulation bras. The former flatten your breasts against your chest, while encapsulation bras are designed to hold each breast separately. Try on a few to see which feels the most comfortable—if you're larger than a B cup, you'll probably want an encapsulation bra, which provides more support. Make sure that the seams don't rub or chafe; washing the bra before wearing it will make it softer.

action

Walk for 20 minutes three times this week at any pace you like. When you have finished each walk, record your progress in your journal.

 # FEELING GOOD

breathing for relaxation

From the moment we take our first inhalation, we do it 24 hours a day, seven days a week, almost always without stopping to think about it. When you breathe, you deliver oxygen to all of your body's cells, including those in your brain. (If you've ever held your breath too long and became light-headed, it's because your brain is starved of oxygen.)

Normal breathing involves deep, slow inhalations and exhalations that start from the very bottom of the lungs. When you're stressed, however, you tend to take shorter, shallower breaths, which fail to use all of your lung capacity, supplying less oxygen to your body and increasing the amount of stress you feel. Yet most people tend to take these short, shallow breaths most of the time. It feels normal because you're so used to it, but chances are you can become a better breather.

Breathing is fundamentally linked to the way we feel, both mentally and physically. The easiest thing you can do to manage stress is to change the way you breathe. Sound too good to be true? When I talk to people about the importance of proper breathing, I get a lot of skeptical looks. Yet deep, slow, focused breathing can change the way you feel, give you an emotional lift, boost your productivity, and reduce stress and anxiety. Once you get in the habit of checking your breathing, you'll find that you can focus and center yourself simply by concentrating on the way you're inhaling and exhaling.

THE FIVE-MINUTE BREATHER You probably can't remember the last time you sat quietly and simply focused on your breath. This five-minute exercise allows you to become aware of your breathing, slows down your heart rate, and reduces your stress levels in the process. It's simple—just sit and be aware of your breathing. Inhale, exhale, and repeat.

Place your hand on your belly as you inhale and exhale. If it barely moves, you're not using much of your lung capacity. As you inhale, your belly should expand, or move outward; as you exhale, it should fall. As you breathe, focus on taking deep, slow breaths in and out, creating more movement in your belly—that means you're using the bottom of your lungs, not just the top.

How do you feel? How does paying attention to your breath change how you feel? You may be surprised how relaxing, energizing, and grounding this small step can be.

action

Your action plan this week is simple: practice the Five-Minute Breathing Exercise once a day. That's it!

week 1 ACTION SUMMARY

 ## eating well

- Stock your pantry with healthy foods, and get used to eating and cooking with healthy ingredients.
- Write down what you eat, and when, in your journal.

 ## getting fit

- Walk for 20 minutes three times this week.
- Note your walks in your journal.

 ## feeling good

- Practice the Five-Minute Breathing Exercise once a day.

WEIGHT

....

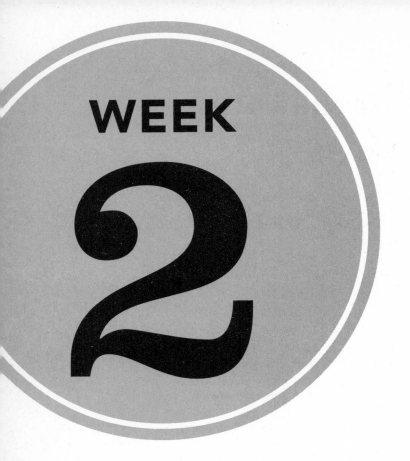

WEEK 2

this week's changes

1. Learn to identify—intuitively—when you are truly hungry, and stop yourself from overeating.

2. Get your three-times-a-week walking program "up to speed."

3. Consider the concept of mindfulness, and begin to be mindful in all aspects of your life.

this week's recipes

Satisfying Soups
- Minestrone Soup
- Creamy Cauliflower Soup
- Savory Butternut Squash Soup
- Vegetable Soup with Pesto

This week you'll learn how to avoid overeating by listening to your body's hunger and satiety signals. These soups can help you get there—research shows that vegetable-based soups are some of the most satisfying foods you can eat, helping fill you up on fewer calories, not to mention packing in important nutrients.

minestrone soup

SERVES 6 *A cup of this chunky soup at the start of a meal just may be a perfect appetite appeaser. A bowl of it with some whole-grain bread and a salad makes a hearty meal.*

- 2 tablespoons olive oil
- 1 large onion, diced
- 2 garlic cloves, minced
- 4 carrots, diced
- 2 stalks celery, diced
- ½ teaspoon dried basil
- ½ teaspoon dried oregano
- 28-ounce can of crushed tomatoes
- 48-ounce can of low-sodium chicken broth or vegetable broth
- 1 cup canned kidney beans, preferably low-sodium, drained and rinsed
- ¾ cup elbow macaroni or other small pasta, such as shells or orzo
- Salt and freshly ground black pepper to taste
- Grated Parmesan cheese (optional)

1. Heat the oil in a large stockpot over a medium flame. Add the onion and cook until soft, about 5 minutes. Lower the heat to low-medium. Add the garlic, carrots, and celery, and cook for about 10 minutes more, or until the vegetables are tender, stirring occasionally. Add a bit of water if the mixture gets too dry while cooking. Add the basil and oregano, and stir to combine.

2. Add the tomatoes and chicken broth, and bring to a boil. Lower the heat to low-medium, add the beans and macaroni, and let simmer for 15 minutes. Season with salt and pepper to taste. Garnish with a sprinkle of Parmesan cheese if desired.

Calories 238; Fat 6.9 g (Sat 1.5 g, Mono 3.6 g, Poly .9 g); Protein 10.3 g; Carb 36.8 g; Fiber 7.8 g; Chol 3.8 mg; Sodium 455 mg

creamy cauliflower soup

SERVES 6 *It always amazes me how a few humble ingredients can be pulled together so easily to yield such a rich, enticing soup. This is a delightfully different and belly-warming way to get your vegetables.*

1 large head cauliflower
1 tablespoon olive oil
1 medium onion, sliced (about 1 cup)
2 medium potatoes, diced (about 1½ cups)
6 cups low-sodium chicken broth or vegetable broth
Salt and freshly ground black pepper to taste
Nutmeg to taste

1. Cut the hard stem out of the cauliflower and break up the head into small florets.

2. In a soup pot, heat the olive oil over a low-medium flame. Add the onion, reduce the heat to low, and cook until golden brown, about 10 minutes, stirring occasionally. Stir in the potatoes. Add the cauliflower and broth, and bring to a boil over a medium heat. Lower the heat to low and let simmer until the cauliflower is very tender, about 20 minutes. Add salt and pepper to taste.

3. Transfer to a blender or use a hand blender and puree until smooth. Sprinkle lightly with nutmeg before serving.

Calories 102; Fat 2.9 g (Sat .4 g, Mono 1.8 g, Poly .4 g); Protein 6.5 g; Carb 14.2 g; Fiber 6 g; Chol 0 mg; Sodium 410 mg

savory butternut squash soup

SERVES 4 *This aromatic, autumnal soup gives you creamy satisfaction, creamlessly. It also provides loads of the antioxidant beta-carotene, which gives the vegetable its brilliant orange hue.*

- 1 tablespoon olive oil
- 1 medium onion, chopped
- 2 garlic cloves, minced
- ¼ teaspoon ground allspice
- ¼ teaspoon ground ginger
- 4 cups cubed butternut or other winter squash, fresh or frozen (about 1½ pounds)
- 4 cups low-sodium chicken broth or vegetable broth
- ¾ teaspoon salt
- 1 tablespoon pure maple syrup
- 4 teaspoons plain low-fat yogurt for garnish (optional)

1. Heat the oil over medium heat in a 6-quart stockpot. Add the onion and cook until soft but not brown, about 6 minutes. Add the garlic, allspice, and ginger, and cook, stirring frequently, for 1 minute more.

2. Add the squash, broth, and salt, and bring to a boil. Reduce heat to medium-low, and simmer until squash is tender and the broth is slightly reduced, about 15 minutes for fresh squash and 5 minutes for frozen.

3. Remove from heat and stir in maple syrup. Allow to cool slightly, about 15 minutes, and then puree with an immersion blender or in a regular blender, about 1 cup at a time, until smooth. Ladle into serving bowls and garnish with yogurt if desired.

Calories 170; Fat 5 g; (Sat 1 g, Mono 3.16 g, Poly .75 g); Protein 7 g; Carb 30 g; Fiber 4 g; Chol 0 mg; Sodium 520 mg

vegetable soup with pesto

SERVES 6 *Herb-infused and chock-full of green and white summer vegetables, this flavorful soup makes for a starter that is both hearty and elegant. Feel free to substitute any green vegetables you may have on hand, from asparagus to broccoli to snow peas.*

2 tablespoons olive oil

1 medium onion, diced

2 stalks of celery, diced

1 medium white or red potato (6 ounces), peeled and cut into ½-inch dice

1 medium zucchini (about 8 ounces), diced

¼ pound green beans (about 20), trimmed and cut into ¾-inch pieces

2 garlic cloves, minced

1 teaspoon fresh thyme leaves, chopped, or ¼ teaspoon dried thyme

¾ teaspoon salt, plus more to taste

½ teaspoon freshly ground black pepper, plus more to taste

6 cups low-sodium chicken broth

1 cup green peas, fresh or frozen

1 tablespoon fresh lemon juice

2 tablespoons store-bought or homemade basil pesto

1. Heat the oil in a large soup pot over a medium-high heat. Add the onion and cook, stirring until it is translucent, about 3 minutes. Lower the heat to medium, add the celery and potato, cover, and cook, stirring occasionally until they begin to soften, about 3 minutes. Add a tablespoon or two of water to the pot if the vegetables begin to stick.

2. Stir in the zucchini, green beans, garlic, thyme, ¾ teaspoon salt, and ½ teaspoon pepper, and cook, stirring occasionally until the vegetables are crisp but beginning to soften, about 3 minutes more

3. Add the chicken broth, bring to a boil, and then reduce heat to medium-low and simmer for 5 minutes, until the vegetables are tender. Stir in the peas and the lemon juice, and then season with additional salt and pepper to taste.

4. To serve, ladle about 1½ cups of the soup into each bowl, and gently stir in about ½ teaspoon pesto until dissolved.

Calories 170; Fat 9 g; (Sat 2 g, Mono 5.4 g, Poly 1 g); Protein 9 g; Carb 17 g; Fiber 3 g; Chol 0 mg; Sodium 420 mg

EATING WELL

understanding hunger

I once asked a friend if she was hungry, and she answered, "What time is it?" Her reply was more profound than she realized, because it had nothing to do with actual hunger. She, like many people, had trained herself to disregard her true hunger and instead relied on the clock to tell her when to eat.

By tuning out real feelings of physical hunger, we shut out one of our body's most basic messages, meant to be signals to satisfy a fundamental need. And by denying true hunger, we also open ourselves up to ignoring the other side of the hunger—satiety, or the sense of feeling full. Once we start eating, we often don't know when to stop, and as a result, we lose one of our most basic weight-management tools.

People overeat all the time simply because the food is there, because it is a good value to buy the "larger" item, or because a dining partner is still eating. Whatever the reason, the underlying problem is that we are ignoring our body's signal that it has had enough.

EATING LIKE A BABY We all come with a built-in hunger-satiety system. To see how well it works, just watch the way a baby eats. When infants are hungry, they demand food and eat enthusiastically. They may pause to rest awhile, eat some more, then gradually stop. You cannot force-feed infants. When they have had enough, they simply stop.

As we get older, this connection with our true hunger and satiety is often drowned out by other food cues we are bombarded with every day. As children, some of us got gold stars for "cleaning our plates"; we learned to associate ham-burgers, hot dogs, chips, ice cream, cake, and candy—all filled with fat, sugar, and/or additives and preservatives—with carefree summer picnics, birthday parties, and other happy occasions. Food companies throughout the world spend millions every year to make our mouths water in advertisements for such items as finger-lickin' chicken, double-crust pizzas, and sugar-laden sodas. After we've been seduced by these cultural signals and have gained too much weight, we go on highly restrictive diets, which only cause us to get further out of touch with our true feelings of physical hunger and satiety. And on it goes.

The good news is that you can get back to that fundamental, baby-like place of eating intuitively. When you do, not only will you have the fuel you need to be energized throughout the day, you will also be healthier—and, if need be, thinner.

EATING INTUITIVELY Take a look at the Hunger Continuum, below. It represents the relative degrees of hunger, starting with 1, for famished, something few of us ever experience, and progressing through 10 for painfully stuffed, which is the sensation of being so full that we might actually feel ill. The goal is to stay in the center of this scale, between 3 and 7, throughout the day. To do this you have to listen to your body—to identify when you are truly, physically hungry. Not bored hungry, lonely hungry, or stressed-out hungry, but truly, stomach-growling hungry. And you have to know when you are satisfied. It takes some practice, but once you tap into these cues, you will have discovered the most natural form of portion control.

hunger continuum

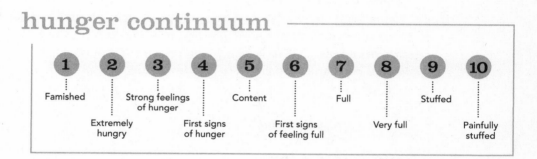

Ideally, you want to eat only when you are truly hungry. If you find yourself reaching for food for reasons besides true hunger, ask yourself why. It may be because you have a designated lunch hour and need to eat at that time, or because you are making an effort to eat breakfast. That is fine. It is not always logistically possible to eat according to your hunger, and it is a good idea to maintain a basic eating schedule—and one that includes breakfast. (I'll get more into that next week.) But beyond that, try not to eat unless you are physically hungry. And don't start eating when you get your first little hunger signals—a bit of hunger is good. It means your body is starting to tap into your fat stores for energy. When your hunger is stronger, but not overwhelming, say at level 3, your body's cues should not be ignored. Then it is time to eat.

KNOWING WHEN TO STOP EATING The opposite end of the spectrum of knowing when you feel physically hungry is knowing when to stop eating. It is important to quit when you experience your first signs of fullness, at about 6 on the Hunger Continuum. All of us have had the experience of eating a delicious meal and reaching a point where we say to ourselves, "I could stop now," but the food is so good that we keep on eating. That is *precisely* the point where we must stop. Most of us are so used to eating way beyond the satiety point that stopping may feel odd at first. However, remind yourself that 20 minutes after you stop eating, once your stomach sensors have had time to tell your brain you are satisfied, you will feel comfortably full and energized, not sleepy and sluggish, the way you feel after you have overeaten.

The key to recognizing this seemingly magical satiety point is to eat slowly, chew each bite, and stop periodically to check in with yourself and note how you are feeling. Slowing down, in particular, works wonders. You will find that you not only eat less, you will enjoy your food more. (You don't really taste your food if you are shoveling it in.) Best of all, your digestion—and your overall health—will improve.

Once you tap into eating intuitively and respond to your hunger-satiety cues, you will find it easier to leave food on your plate. You will also see that portion control doesn't have to be a painstaking chore; instead, you will discover that it really is innate in each of us—if you are only willing to listen to your body.

IS YOUR HUNGER PHYSICAL OR EMOTIONAL? Another reason some of us have problems determining true physical hunger is that we confuse physical hunger with "emotional hunger" or other feelings that we try to satisfy by eating. Deciding whether you are physically hungry or, in fact, emotionally hungry can be tricky and requires some concentration and awareness. Simply pausing for a moment before reaching for food and asking yourself the true nature of your hunger can help.

As a society, we have learned to eat for all sorts of reasons other than physical hunger. We eat "for joy," such as to celebrate an event, like a wedding, birthday, or holiday. We eat because we think we "deserve it," we've had a rough day at work, we finally cleaned out the garage, or even because we walked a mile! We eat because we're sad, from a bit depressed to grieving. We eat because we've just met the love of our lives; we eat because we're lonely. We eat because we're stressed out, overworked, or overwhelmed; we eat because we're bored or tired.

Melissa had been overweight since she was a teenager. She's what I call an "emotional eater." While she ate a fairly healthy diet, she turned to sweets—cookies, cake, brownies, and chocolate—when she was feeling anxious, or lonely, or depressed. She was so used to using food as a comfort, I wasn't surprised that she was struggling with her weight. She wanted to lose at least 40 pounds but struggled with what she called her "obsession" with sugary foods.

Melissa needed to treat food as a fuel for her body, and as one of life's pleasures, rather than as a source of emotional support. I suggested she keep a detailed food

is "cleanse" a dirty word?

We're talking about knowing when to stop eating, so it's a perfect time to mention the latest diet trend: "cleansing," which is basically a form of fasting. Proponents of cleansing say it can produce quick weight loss or jump-start a more realistic eating plan, but I recommend you avoid cleanses for several reasons:

- Cleanses strictly limit what you eat and drink, robbing your body of necessary nutrients. On one popular plan, you drink nothing but water, cayenne pepper, maple syrup, and lemon juice, which provides nearly none of the vitamins and minerals you need for good health.

- They can set you up to gain weight. Yes, you lose weight in the short term—cleanses are extremely low in calories, after all—but that's also a problem. When you slash calories too drastically, you lose muscle, your body's metabolism slows, and, when you start eating normally again, you're more likely to gain weight. Besides, when you're starving yourself, you're likely to wind up bingeing.

- Their claims are often false. I've seen ads saying your body can build up pounds of solid waste and that a cleanse will eliminate this, pardon the pun. But your body doesn't need extreme cleansing to get rid of waste. If you eat a diet that includes plenty of fiber (from fruits, vegetables, nuts, legumes, seeds, and whole grains) and water, your digestive processes should function just fine.

- They don't work in the long term. Real change means developing new habits you can maintain for life. That's the whole idea behind small changes adding up to big results! A cleanse doesn't help you learn new habits—instead of honoring your hunger and eating intuitively, during a cleanse you're supposed to ignore it.

- They're potentially dangerous. Research suggests cleanses and other very-low-calorie diets not only set you up for failure but can impact your health. They may lower your immune function and stress your heart if you do them repeatedly.

So, give up the idea of cleansing your body from the inside, and instead focus on giving your body the right amount of healthy, nutritious fuel. You may not lose as much weight in the short term, but you're more likely to shed extra pounds gradually—and for good.

eight ways to feel full faster and eat less

It may come as a surprise what an impact your environment has on what you eat—and how much. Studies have found that factors ranging from the color of the walls of a room to the size of your plate to whether music is played affect how much you consume. By employing a few tricks, you'll wind up eating less without even trying:

1. **Shrink your plate.** You may not have realized but the average sizes of serving bowls, plates, and glasses have gone up over the years. Chances are that what you think of as a cereal bowl holds two or three servings of cereal—and that what you consider a salad plate is what your parents used for their dinners. You can't do much about growing dinnerware, but you can choose to use smaller sizes when eating at home. Try using a smaller dinner plate, or even a salad plate, for meals—it tricks your eye into thinking you're eating more food than you are, so you wind up just as satisfied but eat smaller portions.

2. **Pack your plate with vegetables.** Foods that pack a lot of fiber and water (think veggies!) fill you up fast without a lot of calories. Aim to fill half your plate with vegetables at each meal. You'll up your nutrient intake and feel fuller, too.

3. **Start with soup.** Soup is filling and takes time to eat—it is linked to weight loss, too. Studies show that people who start their meal with a broth-based soup, especially a chunky one, eat less at the meal and take in fewer calories throughout the day. (Make sure that you skip cream-based soups, as they are high in calories and saturated fat.)

4. **Think small.** The more food you put on your plate (or the more you are served), the more you will eat. Don't heap food onto your plate. Instead, take a modest portion, and go back for seconds after 10 minutes only if you're still truly hungry.

5. Buy small. Package size matters—research shows that people eat more when they're given a bigger food package. So always choose the smallest size package available—or buy the big bag and portion out your own minibags at home.

6. Slow it down. Listening to fast-paced music makes you munch more quickly. Opt for tunes at a slower tempo (or better yet, no music at all).

7. Turn it off. It doesn't matter whether you're watching television, reading the news online, or listening to the radio—eating while doing anything else makes you likely to consume more. Make eating its own activity; you'll enjoy your food more and feel more satisfied, as well.

8. Make the driver's seat a no-food zone. Gobbling food while you're driving can lead to overeating, and it may distract you from what's going on around you. If you must snack on the road, stick to easy-to-eat, portion-controlled snacks like a small bag of nuts or a piece of fruit.

journal, describing not only what she was eating but how she was feeling. "I'd never realized how much I used food as a crutch until I saw it on the page," says Melissa, 37. "If I had a bad day at work or was upset about something, I would automatically soothe myself with a big slice of cake or a frosted brownie. When I was feeling good, I didn't even think about 'junk' food."

It took Melissa time to learn how to manage her feelings without automatically turning to food. "I still crave sweets when I'm feeling bad," she admits today. "But now that I'm aware of it, I try to figure out what's bothering me instead of just reaching for something sweet." She's lost 20 pounds so far and is proud of being able to break her cycle of using food for comfort.

Emotional hunger—the desire to eat even though you're not truly hungry—is most often associated with negative feelings, such as anger, loneliness, frustration, and fear. It's frequently characterized by depression and hopelessness, and is common among women. If you find that you are reaching for food to satisfy these sorts of feelings, try talking with a friend or your spouse, or write in your journal, to get at what's bothering you. If you experience emotional hunger frequently or are unable to curb it, consider one-on-one help from a psychologist and/or registered dietitian or join a local support group.

EATING OUT OF HABIT Another kind of emotional hunger results from old habits, especially the pleasant ones that are associated with feelings of comfort and security. (Eating regular meals and snacks is also a habit, but it is a good one, as I'll explain next week.)

Some of you remember coming home from school, and there would be a glass of milk and a couple of cookies waiting for you. Maybe you weren't really hungry, but your mother was using food as a way to mark the end of the school day and to tide you over until dinner. And wasn't it nice? Didn't you feel loved and cared for?

Many of us have transmuted this kind of old, comforting gesture into a not-so-good adult habit. We use food as a way to separate one part of the day from another or one activity from another. We're finished vacuuming, so we head for the refrigerator; we've walked for 20 minutes, so we reach into the cookie jar. The moment we arrive home from work, we have a beverage or crackers. Most of the time, we aren't hungry; it's just a habit—and it feels good.

The first step to coping with emotional hunger is simply to be aware that you are not physically hungry but are using food to satisfy some other need. The next step is to substitute food with some other activity to deal more constructively with the feelings. For example, if you are eating out of stress, do the Five-Minute Breathing Exercise, take a warm bath, or go for a brisk walk. If you're feeling sad or lonely, don't turn to ice cream—instead, call a friend, write a letter, or write in your journal. If you need a reward for working hard, buy yourself some music, a nice candle, or some scented soap, or treat yourself to a massage instead of rewarding yourself with food.

action

Every time you eat something, register your level of hunger when you begin and your level of satiety when you finish, based on the Hunger Continuum, page 61. Note these levels in your journal. Try to stay between 3 and 7. If you like, also record any feelings of emotional hunger. What are the feelings? Loneliness, anger, frustration, fear, boredom, fatigue? What did you do about the feelings? How often do you experience them?

 # GETTING FIT

walking with purpose

For Week 1, the object was quite simply to get you moving on a regular basis. Now that you've been walking regularly for one week, you are ready to take your regimen to a slightly higher level.

HOW HARD SHOULD YOU EXERCISE? Last week you walked for 20 minutes at a comfortable pace at least three times—or you did enough shorter walks to meet this time requirement. How did you feel? You probably noticed that you felt less stressed afterward—perhaps you were even in a better mood. If you haven't exercised before, consider yourself introduced to regular workouts. Making the commitment and making the time—that's all there is to exercise.

Not all exercise is created equal, however. In general, the more challenging a workout feels, the more benefits you can reap from it. But that doesn't mean you have to suffer to be fit—so you can forget the old "no pain, no gain" theory. It's true that you can't just saunter along for 20 minutes three times a week and expect to radically change your health. You do need to push yourself a little bit to get fitter—what I call exercising along the edge, where you feel that you're challenging yourself but you're not in agony or in pain.

When you're beginning an exercise program, however, you want to up the ante *gradually*. There are several ways to make a workout more challenging: you can do it for a longer period of time; you can exercise more frequently (say, five days a week instead of three); you can increase the intensity at which you exercise.

In this chapter, we'll focus on the third element—intensity. With this program, you'll use three different levels of intensity:

- Level 1, low-intensity walking—relatively slow yet purposeful walking. This type of exercise helps to build stamina and cardiovascular strength, and serves as an excellent fitness walk for beginners. Low-intensity walkers average about three miles per hour and cover one mile in about 20 minutes. This is the level of walking we will focus on for the next few weeks of this program.

- Level 2, mid-intensity walking—a brisker-paced walk where the walker typically moves at about four miles per hour, covering a mile in about 15 minutes. We will reach this level of walking at Week 6 of this program.

- Level 3, high-intensity walking—very fast walking that may include periods of jogging or running; at this level, walkers zip along at about five miles per hour, covering a mile in about 12 minutes. This form of walking is great for burning calories and shaping muscles. We will get to this level at Week 10.

For the next few weeks, you'll maintain the same basic workout plan of walking three days a week, for 20 minutes each time. To make the walk more challenging, you'll focus on its intensity, or how hard your body is working, and start to push yourself—you're going to begin to "walk harder."

FINDING THE RIGHT INTENSITY There are a number of ways to help determine the intensity of any workout. One of the most common uses your heart rate to track how fast your heart is beating during exercise. The faster your heart beats, the harder your body is working. (You've probably seen people at the park or gym taking their pulse during or after exercise—they're measuring their heart rate.)

You may find it helpful to determine a range of heart rates that reflects the level at which you wish to work. This range is called your *target heart rate zone*. Your target heart rate zone is based on your maximum heart rate, or "max," which is the fastest your heart can possibly beat. There are several different formulas used to calculate your max; see Calculating Your Target Heart Rate Zone on page 69 to find your zone for each of the three walking levels.

Once you've determined your target heart rate zone, simply measure your heart rate, or pulse, to ensure that you are walking at the right intensity. To measure your heart rate during exercise, slow down to a comfortable pace, and then place your index and middle fingers at the pulse point on your wrist or at the groove under the left side of your jaw on your neck. Count the number of beats you feel in 15 seconds. Multiply that number by 4 to get the number of beats per minute.

An even easier option is to purchase a heart rate monitor. There are dozens on the market that are accurate, relatively inexpensive, and easy to use. With most, you strap a monitor around your chest, and your heart rate is displayed continuously on a monitor you wear on your wrist. (There are a few models that are worn on your arm, but they may not be as accurate.) Higher-end models let you program in training zones, and an alarm sounds if you begin working too hard (or cheat a little and slow down!). They also include a pedometer function that tells you how far you've walked. The most expensive offer lots of bells and whistles, including the ability to download your workouts to your computer or a GPS (global positioning system) that lets you record how far you walked.

Shopping for a Monitor

Ready to purchase your own monitor? Don't be confused by the wide selection available. There are dozens of models available, but they all fall into three basic types:

- **Continuous-read monitors**—the simplest and least expensive; the monitor simply displays your heart rate. For many exercisers, this is all you'll need. (Price range: about $30–$60.)

- **Zone monitors**—the most popular version. These allow you to program training zones into the monitor; a chime alerts you if you stray from the zone, so you needn't check your display constantly. Different models have different features—some display both your heart rate and your percentage of max (so you don't have to calculate it); others include an automatic calorie counter, as well. (Price range: about $80–$100.)

- **Downloadable monitors** enable you to download your workout information to your computer post-workout; great for serious athletes and techies. Some include a GPS, which also lets you keep track of how far you've gone, and at what pace. (Price range: about $150–$300)

CALCULATING YOUR TARGET HEART RATE ZONE There are several different methods used to calculate maximum heart rate, or max, but here's one of the most common:

Step 1. Calculate your maximum heart rate.

Your maximum heart rate is 220 minus your age. For example, if you are 40 years old, your maximum heart rate is 220 − 40 = 180 beats per minute.

Step 2. Find your target heart rate zone.

- At Level 1, low-intensity walking, the target heart rate zone is 50% to 60% of your maximum heart rate. Multiply your maximum heart rate by .5 and then by .6—your low-intensity zone falls between the two numbers.

For example: for a 40-year-old walking at Level 1, low intensity: 180 x .5 = 90 and 180 x .6 = 108. The target heart rate zone is 90 to 108 beats per minute.

- For Level 2, mid-intensity walking, your target heart rate zone is 60% to 70% of your maximum. Multiply your maximum heart rate by .6 and .7 to find your mid-intensity zone.

- For Level 3, high-intensity walking, your target heart rate zone is 70% to 90% of your maximum. Multiply your maximum heart rate by .7 and .9 to find your high-intensity zone.

Measuring your heart rate is certainly a useful way to calculate the intensity of your exercise, but sometimes all those numbers can make your head spin! Personally, I like to use a scale called the Perceived Exertion Scale below, which is designed to estimate the intensity of exercise based on how you feel as you are working out. It correlates very well with the target heart rate zone formula, so feel free to use either one—or both.

perceived exertion scale

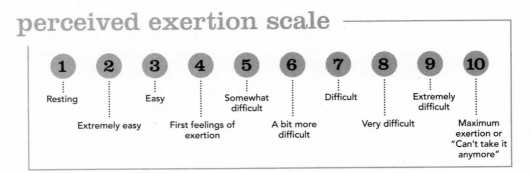

On the Perceived Exertion Scale, low-intensity walking corresponds to a rating of 5 or 6, so walking should feel more purposeful than a mere stroll. Mid-intensity walking corresponds to a 6 or 7 rating and should feel like work, but not enough to exhaust you. And high-intensity walking at 7 to 9 should feel somewhere between challenging and extremely strenuous.

The talk test is another easy way to gauge exercise intensity. By talking aloud as you walk (or run), you can get a general idea of how hard you are working out. For low-intensity walking, you should be able to carry on a conversation, albeit a rather breathy one, with a walking partner. Later, as you graduate to walks of greater intensity and duration, you may be able to speak only in snatches and ultimately be able only to get out a word or two, when you are working your hardest.

action

Your goal this week is similar to last week's—to walk 20 minutes three times. But now I'd like you to begin to pay attention to your pace. Your walks should take some effort and you should feel like you are exerting yourself, but they should not be very difficult, at Level 1, low intensity. Also try speeding up your pace a few times to push yourself a little harder—you'll start to get a feel for what medium-intensity exercise is like. If you are already in the habit of walking regularly and Level 1 feels too easy, bring it up to Level 2 here, pushing yourself a bit more, walking faster than your usual pace.

 # FEELING GOOD

BECOMING MINDFUL I mentioned mindfulness as a core element of wellness in the introduction, and I can't emphasize enough how profoundly this simple concept can improve your quality of life. For me personally, mindfulness is my anchor to a calm, steady, and focused way of being, even when life is at its most hectic.

At its most simplistic, mindfulness is being fully aware of your present moment. When you are being mindful, you are not judging or reflecting—you're not even really thinking. You are simply observing the moment in which you find yourself. When you are being mindful, you have no other purpose than being awake and aware of that moment.

Mindfulness is both simple and complex. In Buddhist thought, it is an integral part of deep meditation and takes years, even lifetimes, to understand fully. At the same time, it can be experienced, in a simple yet effective way, by anyone at any moment.

This week you'll begin to experiment with mindfulness—just for a moment once a day. Instead of listening to the ever-present mental chatter most of us have running through our heads—"We need milk," "What should I make for dinner tonight?," "What's the stock market going to do next?," "I hope my job is safe with all the cutbacks lately," "This place is a pigsty!"— simply stop and focus on the present moment.

Check in with your physical body. How do you feel? Are you feeling energetic, alert, tense, anxious? Or tired, relaxed, sleepy, overwhelmed? What thoughts are racing through your head? Take a few minutes to sit and simply let yourself become aware of your surroundings and your body, without judgment. A good time to do this might be toward the end of the afternoon at work, or while sitting in traffic, or even after dinner.

If you are having trouble quieting your mind, use the Five-Minute Breathing Exercise you have been practicing for the past week. Traditionally, focusing on the breath, as you have been, has been used as a path to mindfulness.

Your mindful moment can be a good time for you to reflect and be thankful. It's easy to get distracted by the things that are "wrong" in our lives—jobs we don't enjoy, conflicts with our loved ones, financial pressures, worries about what's happening in the world today. But I find that stopping and simply focusing on a few things that I'm grateful for calms me and puts me in a more positive frame of mind. It could be something as simple as the fact that the sun is shining, or because my daughter is giggling with happiness, or I had a great night's sleep. Try counting your blessings the next time you feel overwhelmed or irritable—you'll be amazed at how much you have to be thankful about.

EXERCISING MINDFULLY You can approach any activity in a mindful way, and that includes exercise. Mind-body exercise types (think yoga and Pilates) are fast-growing workout trends. Mind-body exercise integrates the physical with the emotional/spiritual to add another layer to your workout; the focus isn't only on what you're doing with your body but what is going through your brain, as well.

You can turn any workout into a more mindful one. For example, as you're walking, don't try to think about all the things you have to do, or that you wish you were anywhere but on that treadmill or pacing around that track. Instead of wishing the moment away or counting the minutes until you're finished, relish it. Get in touch with your body. Notice how your muscles feel, how you may start off stiff but gradually begin to move more fluidly. Notice how your body is breathing deeply, and how good it feels to get your circulation going. Feel your arms swinging in cadence, how your foot lands, grounding you, before you take the next step. If you are outdoors, observe the trees, the sky, the water—whatever makes up your environment. Be in the moment.

eating mindfully

When working with groups and individuals, I have often used this classic meditation exercise. Each participant takes one raisin and concentrates on the experience of eating it—from first enjoying its texture and aroma to gradually chewing and savoring the taste. When they stop to focus on this exercise, people are always amazed at how much flavor is contained in one tiny fruit and how many sensations arise from it.

One of the goals of the exercise is to teach you to slow down and really appreciate food and all its sensory properties. The frenzy of everyday life often leads us to gobble down our food mindlessly. But thoughtless, speedy eating isn't satisfying and can cause overeating and digestive problems. The next time you sit down to a meal, try these exercises, and encourage your family and friends to participate.

- **Say grace.** Offering thanks—to God or whomever you wish to thank—not only for the delicious food but the abundance we enjoy, calms you and focuses your mind on the activity.

- **Consider the food.** Instead of grabbing for your fork, enjoy the aroma and look of the food before you begin to eat—take in all of its sensory pleasure.

- **Eat slowly.** You don't need to chew each bite 40 times, but do savor each bite, chewing slowly. Experience the food's complex and subtle flavors.

- **Pay attention.** Even when you are eating on the go, find a moment to focus mindfully on your eating experience. You'll feel more satisfied if you concentrate on your food instead of trying to work, read, or watch television while you eat.

action

Take at least one moment each day to stop and focus on the present moment, to be mindful.

week 2 ACTION SUMMARY

 ### eating well

- Shop once this week to keep your pantry stocked with healthy foods.
- Stay between 3 and 7 on the Hunger Continuum (see page 61), and register your hunger and satiety levels in your journal each time you eat.
- Maintain your food journal.

 ### getting fit

- Walk for 20 minutes three times at Level 1, low-intensity, or Level 2, mid-intensity.
- Note your walks in your journal.

WEIGHT

....

 ### feeling good

- Do the Five-Minute Breathing Exercise.
- Practice mindfulness at least once a day, perhaps at dinnertime before you begin your meal or just after your walk.

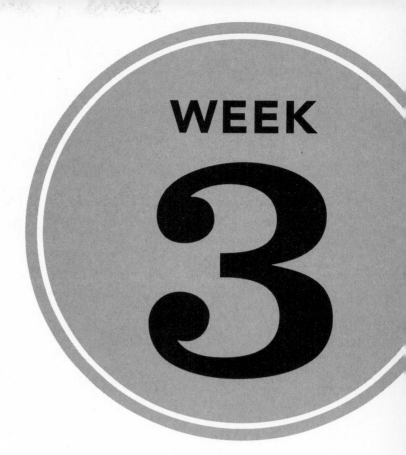

WEEK 3

this week's changes

1. Eat three small meals and one or two snacks daily.

2. Add stretching to your walking regimen.

3. Learn how to manage your time according to your priorities.

this week's recipes

Better Breakfasts

- Banana–Peanut Butter Smoothie
- Strawberry Smoothie
- Cherry Pecan Granola
- Apple Crunch Oatmeal
- Oatmeal 5 Ways
- Whole-Grain Blueberry Pancakes
- Hearty Multigrain Gluten-Free Pancakes

There is no more important meal than breakfast to get you on track for this week's Eating Well change of establishing a healthy, regular eating pattern. Whether you need your breakfast quick and on the go or you have a little more time to relax, I have you covered here with delicious recipes to get you started on the right foot.

banana–peanut butter smoothie

SERVES 1 *The protein-rich combo of peanut butter and yogurt makes this smoothie especially satisfying and will give you the lasting energy you need to get through the morning. Pour it into a to-go cup and drink it on your way out the door if time is tight.*

1 cup nonfat vanilla yogurt
1 medium banana
1 tablespoon smooth, natural-style peanut butter
1 cup ice

Put all the ingredients into a blender and blend until smooth.

Calories 363; Fat 8.7 g (Sat 1.9 g, Mono 3.9 g, Poly 2.3 g); Protein 14.2 g; Carb 60.7 g; Fiber 3.8 g; Chol 0 mg; Sodium 211 mg

strawberry smoothie

SERVES 1 *Mix it up and substitute any kind of berry, mango, cherries, or peaches in this frothy treat. For extra fiber and nutrients, try adding a tablespoon of wheat germ, as well.*

1 cup frozen strawberries (about 6 berries)
½ cup nonfat vanilla yogurt
½ cup nonfat milk
¼ cup ice water

Put all the ingredients into a blender and blend until smooth.

Calories 166; Fat .7 g (Sat .2 g, Mono .1 g, Poly .3 g); Protein 9.5 g; Carb 31.0 g; Fiber 3.3 g; Chol 2.4 mg; Sodium 133 mg

cherry pecan granola

SERVES 10 *You can make this granola with any combination of chopped nuts and dried fruit you like or happen to have on hand. Enjoy it on yogurt, with milk, or to add crunch to oatmeal. It is so simple to make and so much better than anything you can find in a package.*

    Cooking spray
 2 cups old-fashioned rolled oats
 ¾ cup coarsely chopped, unsalted pecans
 ⅓ cup pure maple syrup
 ½ tablespoon canola oil
 ½ teaspoon vanilla extract
 ¼ teaspoon ground cinnamon
 ⅛ teaspoon salt
 ⅓ cup dried cherries

1. Preheat the oven to 300°F. Coat a baking sheet with cooking spray.

2. In a large bowl combine the oats, pecans, maple syrup, oil, vanilla, cinnamon, and salt until evenly coated. Spread on the baking sheet and bake until golden brown, stirring occasionally, about 30 minutes. Transfer the sheet to a wire rack, and allow to cool completely. Stir in the cherries. Store in an airtight container in the refrigerator for up to 2 weeks.

Calories 170; Fat 8 g; (Sat. 5 g, Mono 2.7 g, Poly 2 g); Protein 4 g; Carb 22 g; Fiber 3 g; Chol 0 mg; Sodium 30 mg

apple crunch oatmeal

SERVES 1 *There are so many delicious ways to dress up oatmeal. This is one of my favorites, especially in the fall after going apple picking.*

1 cup nonfat milk
½ cup old-fashioned rolled oats
½ cup diced and peeled apple
2 teaspoons packed dark brown sugar
2 tablespoons granola

1. Put the milk, oats, and apple into a saucepan over a medium-high flame and, stirring frequently, bring to a boil. Reduce the heat to low and, stirring occasionally, cook for about 5 minutes or until the oatmeal reaches the consistency you like.

2. Transfer the oatmeal mixture to a cereal bowl. Stir in the brown sugar and top with the granola.

Calories 354; Fat 4.4 g (Sat .8 g, Mono 1 g, Poly 1.4 g); Protein 15 g; Carb 65.3 g; Fiber 6.3 g; Chol 5 mg; Sodium 161 mg

oatmeal 5 ways

Prepare your oatmeal with milk or soy milk instead of water to add protein, minerals, and vitamins. Regular oats are well worth the 5 minutes of cooking time, but if you.need to, you can use quick-cooking oatmeal instead.

pumpkin spice • Stir in a dollop of canned pumpkin puree, plus a sprinkle of ginger, nutmeg, cinnamon, and brown sugar.

strawberry swirl • Add sliced fresh berries, or thawed frozen strawberries with their juice, to your cooked oatmeal. Then swirl in a little strawberry jam for sweetness.

fruit and nut • Add chopped dried apricots, dried plums, and raisins to your oatmeal as it is cooking so that the fruit plumps up a little. Then add some toasted, chopped walnuts and almonds, and a touch of honey.

banana walnut • Top your cooked oatmeal with sliced bananas, chopped toasted walnuts, and a bit of honey.

oatmeal cookie • Add all the flavors that make oatmeal cookies so good: a drop of vanilla extract, some raisins, cinnamon, and a little brown sugar.

whole-grain blueberry pancakes

SERVES 4 *These hearty pancakes are a big treat on the weekends when you have a little more time to prepare breakfast. You can also make the batter the night before and store it in the refrigerator.*

¾ cup whole wheat flour
½ cup all-purpose flour
¼ cup cornmeal
2 tablespoons wheat germ
2 teaspoons sugar
2 teaspoons baking powder
½ teaspoon baking soda
¼ teaspoon salt
2 large eggs
¾ cup skim milk
1 cup low-fat buttermilk
¼ teaspoon pure vanilla extract
1 cup blueberries, fresh or frozen

1. In a medium bowl mix together the dry ingredients (flour through salt). In another bowl, beat together the eggs and skim milk, then stir in the buttermilk and vanilla extract.

2. Preheat a large nonstick griddle or skillet over a medium-low flame. Stir the wet ingredients into the dry ingredients, mixing only enough to combine them. Stir in the blueberries. (If you are using frozen berries, you don't need to defrost them.)

3. Ladle a scant ¼ cup of the batter onto the griddle or skillet. Flip when golden brown on the bottom, 1½ to 2 minutes. Cook the other side until golden brown. Serve immediately, or keep warm in a 200°F oven until the entire batch is ready.

Calories 283; Fat 4.5 g (Sat 1.4 g, Mono 1.3 g, Poly 1 g); Protein 13.1 g; Carb 49.2 g; Fiber 5.1 g; Chol 110 mg; Sodium 626 mg

hearty multigrain gluten-free pancakes

SERVES 4 *Even if you are not gluten intolerant, chances are that at some point you will need to cook for someone who is. (See Get Rid of Gluten? page 197.) No matter, you will enjoy these pancakes just because they taste so good.*

    1 cup brown rice flour
    ¼ cup cornmeal
    1 tablespoon cornstarch
    2 tablespoons ground flax
    2 teaspoons baking powder
    ½ teaspoon table salt
    1 cup low-fat buttermilk
    2 large eggs
    1 tablespoon canola oil
    1 tablespoon honey
    1 teaspoon pure vanilla extract
      Nonstick cooking spray

1. In a large bowl, whisk the brown rice flour, cornmeal, cornstarch, ground flax, baking powder, and salt. In a medium bowl, beat the buttermilk, eggs, oil, honey, and vanilla.

2. Coat a large nonstick griddle or skillet with cooking spray and preheat over medium-low heat. Stir the buttermilk mixture into the flour mixture until combined.

3. Ladle a scant ¼ cup of the batter per pancake onto the griddle or skillet. Flip when golden brown on the bottom, 1½ to 2 minutes.

4. Cook the other side until golden brown, another 1½ minutes. Serve immediately or keep warm in a 200°F oven until the entire batch is ready.

Calories 310; Fat 9 g (Sat 1.5 g, Mono 4 g, Poly 3 g); Protein 9 g; Carb 47 g; Fiber 3 g; Chol 110 mg; Sodium 640 mg

EATING WELL

the optimal eating pattern

For the past week you have been trying to eat more intuitively—waiting till you are physically hungry and stopping when you are satisfied. You probably find you are eating smaller amounts than you did before, and you may be surprised to find how little it takes to make you feel full. Isn't it great not to feel stuffed after dinner?

But, as I mentioned in the last chapter, just as it is important to eat only when you are truly hungry, it is also important to have a basic eating schedule. This week you'll begin to guide your body into an optimal eating pattern—one that will keep you energized all day, help reduce cravings and impulsive eating, and may even help you lower your cholesterol.

The meal pattern that I find works best for most people is three meals and one or two snacks in regular intervals throughout the day. That may sound like a lot, but the key here is keeping those meals and snacks *small*. (See Appendix C, Serving Sizes, on page 294, and Appendix B, Sample Week of Healthy Eating, on page 292.)

At first you may find that eating this frequently goes against your hunger cues. Many people tell me they are not hungry for breakfast, for example, or that they prefer to skip lunch. If that's the case, chances are you have trained your body into the all too common trap of eating little throughout the day and overeating at night. I have counseled dozens of people who regularly have nothing but coffee and some fruit or a bagel all day, only to eat a gargantuan dinner at night. Consuming most of your daily calories in the evening is bad for your digestion, and it deprives your body of fuel when you need it most—during the day. It also sets you up to skip meals again the next day. After all, who is hungry for breakfast after sleeping on a big, heavy dinner?

Jodi was a college student whose mother asked me to talk to her. Jodi was only 21, yet she had trouble concentrating on her classwork and frequently felt exhausted. After I spoke with her, it was easy to identify the problem. She was basically starving herself during the day.

Jodi wanted to lose a few pounds (though she was already at a healthy body weight), so she would skip breakfast and then eat a tiny lunch—maybe an apple or a bag of pretzels. Between classes, she survived on diet soda and coffee. By the time she got home, she was irritable, exhausted, and starving. She would wind up eating pizza with her roommates or polishing off a box of cookies, which made it impossible for her to lose weight.

Though Jodi was a smart young woman, her eating habits were far from smart. After explaining that her body and her brain needed energy during the day, I had her commit to eating breakfast and lunch every day. She was worried that she'd gain weight, but I promised her she'd burn those calories off. Two weeks later, Jodi had already noticed a huge difference not only in her energy level but in her mood. She was able to concentrate better, and even her roommates had commented on how much happier she seemed. Hopefully her new habits will last her a lifetime.

When you start eating more throughout the day and less in the evening, you'll begin to wake up hungry, eager for breakfast. Your stomach will let you know when it's time for lunch. This catches a lot of people off-guard. They feel uncomfortable with that hunger, which may be new to them, and fear it will make them eat more in the long run. But it won't. Research shows that people who skip breakfast usually wind up overeating later in the day, making up for the calories they tried to save, and then some. In fact, people who eat breakfast tend to be leaner than those who skip it. They also perform better on cognitive tests, and they are more likely to satisfy their nutritional needs overall.

One of the main benefits of adopting the three-meals-and-two-snacks pattern is that it keeps your energy high throughout the day. Eating regularly helps stabilize your blood sugar, also known as glucose. When you go too long without eating, your blood sugar dips, and since glucose is the brain's primary fuel, those dips can leave you foggy, fatigued, irritable, and light-headed. You know that crabby, edgy feeling you get when you haven't had lunch and you're quick to snap at your kids or your coworkers? That feeling magically disappears when you eat at regular intervals. As a bonus, research proves that people who eat more frequently have lower total cholesterol and more good cholesterol than people who skip meals!

Eating regularly also helps you eat healthier. Meal skippers are more likely to make impulsive—and often unhealthy—food choices. It's a lot harder to resist those M&Ms on your coworker's desk when your head is spinning from not having eaten all morning. And when you have starved yourself all day, you somehow feel deserving of a few extra pieces of bread slathered with butter and a hunk of chocolate cake at dinner.

Having a set meal pattern also helps prevent the evening haze of constant mindless munching, where dinner has no real end but drags on from one snack to the next until you roll yourself into bed. With a set meal pattern, you stop eating for the day after dinner or a small evening snack. You may want to pick an absolute time to stop eating if nighttime nibbling is an issue for you.

The meal pattern I recommend is three moderate meals (breakfast, lunch, and dinner) and one or two small snacks a day, one mid-morning and one midafternoon. But that pattern isn't the only way to go. Some people prefer to graze, eating six smaller meals throughout the day. Others find it works better for their weekend schedule to eat two meals (brunch and dinner) and two or three snacks.

Whatever pattern you prefer, remember that the midafternoon snack is key. Around three or four o'clock, most people's energy levels start to flag. That's when they reach for the chocolate and caffeine, hoping to summon the energy to exercise or get through the rest of their day. But if you plan to eat a healthy snack at that time, you'll be amazed at how much more stamina you have, how much more you can put into your walks, and how much easier it is to avoid overeating at dinner. You'll also be less likely to inhale whatever's in your refrigerator or pantry when you come home from work, and be willing to take the time to make a healthy dinner.

You may be thinking that you hardly have time to prepare and eat one healthy meal a day, much less three meals plus snacks. But it is not as difficult as it sounds. Look at the 12 Quick High-Energy Snacks below—neither they nor your meals have to be elaborate creations. And, although it is important to sit down to a relaxed meal whenever possible, it is perfectly fine (and often necessary) to eat on the go. With the pantry you established in Week 1 and a little prep work, you have plenty of options that will keep you going when time is tight.

If you haven't done so already, make sure you have on hand individual-size servings of tuna, yogurt, yogurt drinks, low-fat cheese, small boxes of whole-grain cereal, and instant soups. Invest a few minutes each week to prepare foods that you can grab and eat on the go. When you make dinner, make a little extra for the next day. Hard-boil a few eggs. Wash and slice veggies like peppers, celery, and carrots, and store them in a container in the fridge. Keep a supply of healthy foods at work. Stash some nuts and dried fruit in your car. And, if you are at a food court or need to hit the drive-through, go for the healthiest options.

12 QUICK HIGH-ENERGY SNACKS Going too long without eating can make you feel tired, cranky, and spaced-out. Small, healthy snacks or mini-meals that include protein and carbohydrates will help keep your energy levels high throughout the day, and they take little time to prepare. Most of these make a good breakfast on the go, too.

1. Sliced apple with peanut butter or almond butter (1 tablespoon)

2. Turkey (2 slices) and tomato on whole wheat bread (1 slice)

3. Low-fat cottage cheese (½ cup) and a peach or pear

4. A hard-boiled egg and a piece of fruit

5. Almonds (⅓ cup) and dried apricots (¼ cup)

6. A yogurt-and-fruit smoothie (12 ounces) (1½ cups)

7. Hummus (¼ cup) and sliced red bell pepper (1 cup)

8. Low-fat yogurt (1 cup) and fresh strawberries (1 cup)

9. Baked sweet potato (½ potato) with low-fat cottage cheese (½ cup)

10. Baked tortilla chips (10) and bean dip (½ cup)

11. Slice of cheese (1½ ounces) and whole-grain crackers (5)

12. Half a peanut butter and banana sandwich (1 tablespoon peanut butter, 1 piece of whole-grain bread)

High-Energy Eating

If you experience energy slumps throughout the day, it may be your diet that's bringing you down. These energy-boosting tips can help get you back to speed.

- **Don't skip meals.** Skipping meals makes your blood sugar dip and deprives your brain of the fuel it needs to function optimally.

- **Include some protein at each meal.** Protein-rich foods like fish, poultry, lean meat, eggs, beans, nuts, yogurt, milk, and cheese help prevent that sleepy feeling you can get after a meal; they also take longer to digest, so you feel full longer.

- **Avoid sugary foods and refined starches like white bread.** These foods make blood sugar spike quickly and then fall again, causing energy lows.

- **Avoid large, heavy, fatty meals.** They leave you feeling sluggish because your body is working overtime to digest them.

- **Drink plenty of water and other fluids.** Fatigue is one of the first symptoms of dehydration, so drink plenty of water throughout the day to stay energized.

HEALTHY FAST FOOD I probably don't have to tell you that a typical fast food meal can contain a day's worth of saturated fat, salt, and calories, and that much of the food is still highly processed. However, most chains are making efforts to offer healthier alternatives, and though these are not ideal choices, at most places you can now find options that are at least better for you and relatively low-calorie.

If you have more than one fast-food restaurant to choose from, opt for those that serve more than burgers and fries. "Fast casual" restaurants like Panera Bread, Au Bon Pain, Noodles and Company, Corner Bakery Café, and Atlanta Bread all made *Health* magazine's top 10 healthiest fast food restaurants list because of the diversity of their menus. Starbucks also offers quite a few healthy, convenient food options. Many of these restaurants now list the calorie counts directly on their menus, so you can compare options. (If not, remember you can always check their websites for nutrient info on your smartphone while you're waiting in line!)

If you're stuck ordering somewhere that doesn't give you access to nutritional data, think small. If you simply *must* have a burger and fries, get the smallest size possible (and that's usually about the portion you should be consuming anyway).

Ask for sandwiches to be served without mayo or sauce and look for smart, lower-cal choices like these:

- Grilled chicken sandwich
- Salad with grilled chicken (go easy on the dressing)
- Bean burrito
- Turkey, ham, or veggie sub (small size on whole-grain bread)
- Baked potato with broccoli and cheese
- Broth-based soup
- Low-fat yogurt and fruit parfait
- Smoothies made with whole fruit
- Oatmeal with nuts and fruit

action

This week you'll establish a regular eating pattern, eating three meals and one or two snacks a day.

Smarter Fast Food with Your Smartphone

Hitting the drive-through window? Do it smartly. Use one of these apps to get the nutrition facts of your meal before you order:

- Fast Food Calories:
  www.itunes.apple.com/us/app/fast-food-calories

- Fast Food Calorie Counter:
  www.itunes.apple.com/us/app/fast-food-calorie-counter

- Nutrition Facts:
  www.itunes.apple.com/us/app/nutrition-facts

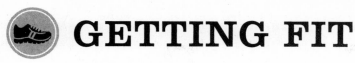

GETTING FIT

stretching

During the last two weeks, you've been walking three times a week. Now we're going to add one simple component to your fitness plan—stretching. It's a basic element of fitness, but one that most of us ignore.

WHY STRETCH? Okay, be honest—when was the last time you felt flexible instead of stiff? At the end of the day, does your back ache or your neck feel stiff and sore? Do you notice little twinges when doing something as minor as bending over to tie your shoes? Unless you do yoga or stretch regularly, you've probably noticed that you're not as flexible as you used to be. While most of us neglect stretching, doing it regularly can help prevent injury, promote flexibility, maintain your range of motion, and serve as a great relaxation tool.

As you grow older, you tend to lose some flexibility, which makes you more likely to suffer an injury. For example, 80% of people suffer from back pain at some point in their lives. Stretching can prevent common injuries and improve your over-all flexibility—in one study, people who stretched for 30 seconds per muscle group each day increased their range of motion significantly in just a few weeks' time.

Taking just a few minutes to stretch several times a week can pay off in the way you feel throughout the day. Perform these simple stretches after warming up or after you've exercised—it's easier and more effective to stretch with nice loose muscles. Stretching when your muscles are cold and stiff, on the other hand, may make you more likely to suffer an injury. One of the simplest ways to incorporate stretching into your routine is to make it part of your cool-down routine.

SIX SIMPLE STRETCHES You don't have to do a backbend or headstand to benefit from stretching. Some of the simplest stretches are the most effective.

Remember to stretch after warming up or exercising when your muscles are looser and more flexible. You want to hold each stretch for three to five breaths. (I like to use breaths rather than counting because it helps you relax into the stretch.) Don't strain or stretch to the point of discomfort, and don't bounce while you're performing these moves. You want to stretch to the "edge"—you should feel a pull in the muscles you're targeting, but it shouldn't be painful.

Finally, don't get discouraged if you can't stretch very far when you begin per-forming these moves. Some people are more flexible than others, and you may progress slowly at first. Simply stretch as far as you can without pain—over time, you will notice an increase in your flexibility.

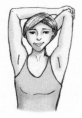

Triceps stretch Stand with your arms over your head. Grasp your left elbow in your right hand and pull it toward your head, with the fingers of your left hand pointing down toward your spine. Feel a comfortable stretch in the back of your shoulder and upper back. Repeat with the arms switched.

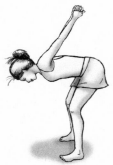

Chest/shoulders/hamstrings stretch Stand and place your hands behind your back, with palms facing each other and fingers clasped. With your feet shoulder width apart, bend your knees slightly and lean forward so that your back is parallel to the floor, gently pulling your arms up toward the ceiling as you do so. When you feel a comfortable stretch in your shoulders and chest, straighten your legs as much as you comfortably can and extend the stretch to your hamstrings, the muscles along the backs of your thighs.

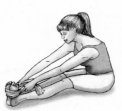

Hamstring stretch Sit on the ground with your legs in front of you. Bend forward and reach toward your toes—grasp them if you can, or hold your shins. (You can also wrap a towel around your feet and hold onto that while you stretch.) Without bending your knees, stretch forward as far as you can—you should feel it in your hamstrings and lower back.

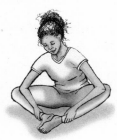

Butterfly stretch (inner thighs) Sit up tall and bring the soles of your feet together, letting your knees drop to the sides. Gently pull your heels toward your body and then press your knees toward the floor until you feel a comfortable stretch along your inner thighs. Grasping your feet with your hands, gently pull yourself forward by bending at the hips. If you want, you can press your elbows down on your legs to increase the stretch.

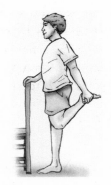

Quadriceps stretch Stand with your hand on a wall or other stationary object for balance. Bend your left leg and hold your left foot behind your body with your left hand; gently pull toward your buttocks. Repeat on the other side with the right leg and hand.

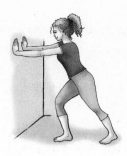

Calf stretch Stand facing a wall two to three feet away. Step your left foot about 18 inches behind you. Keeping your left leg straight, bend your right leg. Lean forward and press against the wall, keeping both heels on the floor—you'll feel the stretch in your left calf. Then repeat on the other side, stepping back with your right foot and stretching the calf muscle of your right leg.

action

Your action plan this week is simple. Continue walking three times a week at a low-to mid-intensity level. After your walk, perform the Six Simple Stretches.

 # FEELING GOOD

managing your time

The number one excuse for not exercising? Lack of time. Today it seems like none of us have enough time to do the things we really want to. Most of us carry around a to-do list a mile long every day and then spend weekends checking tasks off the list, only to have new ones spring up in their place.

There are only 24 hours in a day. If you always feel frazzled and it seems like you're spending all your time doing the things you *have* to do—and no time doing the things you *want* to do—it's time to learn how to manage your time better.

Does the idea of time management bring to mind complicated charts and having to track and account for every possible minute? Relax. You can prioritize and manage your time more efficiently in four simple steps.

STEP 1: TAKE A LOOK AT YOUR LIFE Figure out how you're spending your time. Consider how long you spend doing different activities in a typical day. You needn't account for every single second, but estimate how much time you spend on the activities below. You may find it helpful to track two weekdays and one weekend day for a more accurate picture of how you spend your time. You can record the time here:

ACTIVITY	DAY 1	DAY 2	DAY 3	AVERAGE
Getting showered/dressed/ready in the morning				
Eating breakfast/reading the paper				
Getting your kids ready in the morning (including making breakfast, taking care of lunch money, reminding about homework, driving kids to school, etc.)				
Commuting to work/working				
Preparing/eating lunch				
Preparing/eating dinner (and don't forget doing the dishes!)				
Business-related activities				
Using the Internet/sending and receiving e-mail				
Running errands				
Doing household chores (laundry, cleaning, paying bills, grocery shopping, yard work)				
Child-care tasks (helping kids with homework, playing games, separating dueling siblings, driving to soccer games)				
Watching television				
Reading (newspapers/magazines/books)				
Exercising/sports				
Spending time with your spouse/partner (talking, dinner out, sex, and "couple time")				
Charity/volunteer activities				
Socializing and spending time with friends/family				
Sleeping				
Health/beauty (salon/doctor/dental appointments and the like)				
Hobbies/downtime				
Other activities:				

STEP 2: CONSIDER YOUR PRIORITIES Now make a list of your priorities, in order. (For most people, the order is the tricky part.) Include children, spouse, other family members, friends, your job, your church, community or volunteer activities, exercise, having a clean house, watching a favorite television show, hobbies, sex, and the like. Put them in order as best you can:

my priorities

1 ....
2 ....
3 ....
4 ....
5 ....
6 ....
7 ....
8 ....
9 ....
10 ....

How'd you do? If you struggled with this exercise, you're not alone—most of us have a hard time deciding what's most important. Of course, your kids are your number one priority. But your spouse is important, too! And your parents and siblings. And your friends. And your career. And being financially secure. And having a nice-looking home. And let's not forget—yourself. With all the competing demands on our time, it's no wonder a lot of us feel overwhelmed.

Obviously, some things will be priorities out of necessity. Your job may not be the most significant aspect of your life, but it's the way you put food on the table and provide for yourself and your family. That makes it important. Consider all the factors as you order (and feel free to reorder) what your priorities really are.

STEP 3: COMPARE THE RESULTS Okay, you've done the hardest part. Now take a closer look at the total amounts of time you're spending. How do they correlate to your priorities? If you work, you probably spend more time with your coworkers than your children. That may be unavoidable. But if you spend 12 hours a week watching television and 1 hour exercising—yet you say your "health" is one of your priorities—then it's best to reevaluate how you spend your time. (And by the way, how much time do you spend watching the tube? The average adult watches at least two hours a day, every day. Couldn't those hours be better spent doing something else?)

STEP 4: START MAKING CHANGES With your priority list in hand, look at where you're spending your time, and consider ways that you can change your schedule. Can you group errands into a single two-hour block each week instead of doing them every day? Could you brown-bag your lunch and use the time to catch up on work instead of eating out every afternoon? If you spend hours driving your kids to and fro, could you carpool? Can you limit the television you watch to a few favorite shows instead of zoning out in front of the tube every night? And what about all that time you spend on the computer not doing work? Is it time to cut back on your video games or the amount of time you're on social media?

Check whether you're overextended with your volunteer obligations, as well. It's wonderful to contribute to causes you believe in, but many people overcommit themselves—at their own (and often their family's) expense. Come up with ways you can combine some of your priorities, like making a standing date with a friend to exercise together, so you can get fit while also getting caught up on your lives.

Start incorporating the changes that are important to you into your daily life. It may mean asking your kids or your spouse for help. Are your kids old enough to start helping with household chores? Can your partner take over some of the errands on Saturday morning? Maybe it's better to turn down the chance at overtime to focus on the other aspects of your life right now.

Remember, there will always be urgent tasks—paying bills, running errands, taking the car in to get the oil changed—that must be done. Don't be distracted by those and let your health, relationships, or well-being be the last thing you worry about. We all get the same 24 hours in each day. How you spend it, however, is up to you.

LEARNING TO SAY NO There's one magic word that can change your life, give you back control over your time, and help you lead a happier life. That word is *no*.

But I bet you have trouble saying no, don't you? I can sympathize. You don't want to turn down that committee job for your son's school. Your daughter will be crushed if you're not the parent helper again this year. Your company always relies on you to organize the holiday party. Guess what? Sometimes you have to say no—to protect yourself, your time, and your energy.

But how? *No* seems like a mean word, a selfish word, and you're not selfish, right? I'll make the job easy for you—here are six ways to say no and not feel bad about it:

1. **Say "No, thanks."** Feel bad about saying just "No"? Thank the person for the opportunity before you turn him or her down. "I really appreciate you thinking of me, but no, thank you." See? You can be polite when you're turning people down.

2. **Stall for time.** Too often we agree to do something on the spur of the moment. When asked for something, tell the person you need to think about it and you'll let them know. Then you can decide whether you want to take on the responsibility.

3. **Counter with an alternative.** If you know you're not interested in the job or task but are willing to do something else, say so. "I'm sorry, I can't take on the chair responsibility, but I'm willing to help with the event the day of." (This is mostly a no, but it allows you to participate in something you want to without giving up your life for it.)

4. **Give a reason(s).** Sometimes you have to say no, and you've got a good reason—or 10 of them—for doing so. If you're comfortable sharing them, let the person know—or simply say that you've been overextended lately and need to cut back.

5. **Or don't.** "I'm sorry, but I can't." That's it. That's all you have to say. Yes, you'll feel guilty for a few minutes . . . but think how relieved you'll be afterward.

6. **Suggest someone else.** You can't do it, but you know someone who might be interested? Pass along the person's name—it may be just right for him or her.

action

Your action plan this week is to start taking control of your time and to practice saying no to things that don't fit your priorities.

week 3 ACTION SUMMARY

 ## eating well

- Shop to replenish your healthy pantry.
- Stay between 3 and 7 on the Hunger Continuum (see page 61).
- Eat three meals and one or two snacks each day.
- Maintain your food journal.

 ## getting fit

- Walk for 20 minutes at low to mid intensity, three times.
- Add stretching to your walking routine.
- Note your walks in your journal.

 ## feeling good

- Do the Five-Minute Breathing Exercise daily.
- Practice a moment of mindfulness daily.
- Say no to tasks you don't want to and don't have to do.

WEIGHT
....

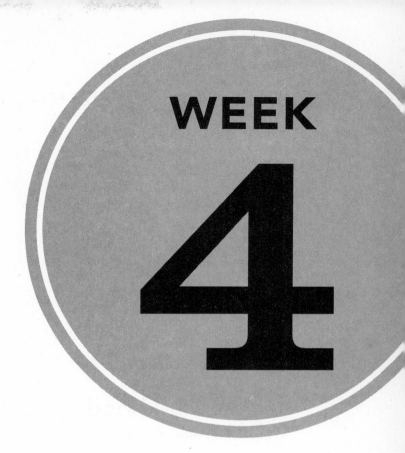

WEEK 4

this week's changes

1. Drink enough water and cut back on sugary drinks.
2. Add strengthening moves to your walking routine.
3. Create a bedtime ritual for better sleep.

this week's recipes

Healthy Thirst Quenchers

- Spa Water
- Pink Cocktail
- Watermelon-Mint Flavored Water
- Ginger Green Iced Tea

This week you will discover why it is important to drink water throughout the day and how much you actually need. You will also focus on eliminating sweetened drinks from your diet. And, while plain water is the ideal hydrator, sometimes you want something more exciting to drink. These healthy drink recipes fit the bill perfectly—they are tasty and thirst-quenching, and also make for a beautiful presentation.

spa water

SERVES 4 *They served this water at a spa I once visited, and I have been making it ever since. It somehow makes water even more refreshing. You can also add a sprig of mint if you have some on hand.*

½ cucumber, peeled and sliced
3 slices of lemon

Put the ingredients in a pitcher with 1 quart of cold water and stir. Allow to sit for at least 20 minutes before serving.

Calories 5; Fat 0 g (Sat 0 g, Mono 0 g, Poly 0 g); Protein 0 g; Carb 1 g; Fiber 1 g; Chol 0 mg; Sodium 10 mg

pink cocktail

SERVES 1 *Order this festive drink at a bar when you want to cut back on alcohol. Just ask for club soda with a splash of cranberry and a wedge of lime.*

1 cup club soda
¼ cup cranberry juice cocktail
1 lime wedge

Pour the club soda over a glass of ice. Add the cranberry juice and a squeeze of lime, and stir.

Calories 37; Fat 0 g; Protein 0 g; Carb 9.6 g; Fiber .1 g; Chol 0 mg; Sodium 51 mg

watermelon-mint flavored water

SERVES 6 *I came up with this recipe in response to my daughter, who was being lured at the grocery store by rows of bottles of brightly colored, flavored water. My tasty, lightly sweetened beverage is a gorgeous pink, has only a fraction of the sugar and none of the artificial dyes found in most of the packaged water drinks, and is a hit with children and adults alike.*

¼ cup lightly packed fresh mint leaves
1 tablespoon granulated sugar
1 cup boiling water
4 cups cubed, seedless watermelon (16 ounces)
2 tablespoons freshly squeezed lime juice

1. Place the mint leaves and sugar in a small pot and pour the boiling water over. Using a wooden spoon, stir until the sugar dissolves; then crush the mint leaves with the spoon to muddle them. Allow to steep and cool for 15 minutes.

2. Meanwhile, place the watermelon and 2 cups of cold water in a blender and puree. Using a fine-mesh strainer, strain the watermelon liquid into a large pitcher; discard the solids.

3. Strain the mint leaves out of the pot and discard them. Add the mint "tea" to the pitcher with the watermelon liquid. Add 2 more cups of cold water and lime juice to the pitcher and stir to combine. Serve over ice.

Calories 30; Fat 0 g; Protein 0 g; Carb 10 g; Fiber 0 g; Chol 0 mg; Sodium 10 mg

ginger green iced tea

SERVES 4 *Ginger and green tea have each been credited with multiple health benefits. Here they come together deliciously in a refreshing summer drink.*

    5 cups water
    2½-inch piece of fresh ginger (unpeeled is okay),
       coarsely chopped
    3 tablespoons honey
    6 bags of green tea
       Mint sprigs (optional)

1. Place 2 cups water and the ginger into a saucepan and bring to a boil. Reduce the heat to low and simmer for 5 minutes. Stir in the honey. Remove the pan from heat and add the tea bags. Steep for 3 minutes, and then strain out all the solids.

2. In a large pitcher combine the strained tea with the remaining 3 cups water. Chill in the refrigerator. Serve over ice, garnished with mint sprigs, if using.

Calories 50; Fat 0 g; Protein 0 g; Carb 13 g; Fiber 0 g; Chol 0 mg; Sodium 10 mg

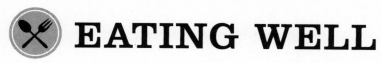

EATING WELL

you are what you drink

When you think "nutrition," the first words that come to mind are likely *vitamins, minerals, carbohydrates, fat,* and *protein*—all important nutrients. But the most vital nutrient is one that is often overlooked: water. For staying healthy and feeling your best, water works wonders. Even slight dehydration can cause fatigue, weakness, dizziness, and headaches. That's why getting enough fluid is a cornerstone of feeling well. But beyond basic hydration, studies show that water can help prevent conditions like kidney stones and cancers of the urinary tract and colon. This week we are going to make sure you are drinking what you need to keep you at the top of your game.

HOW MUCH IS ENOUGH? You have probably heard more than one nutritionist say you should drink eight 8-ounce glasses of water a day. While this advice makes a catchy phrase, it is not completely accurate. Fluid needs are very individual. The amount you personally need depends upon your metabolism, your activity level, and the climate you are in. Plus, there are many beverages besides water that count toward hydration.

According to the National Academy of Sciences Food and Nutrition Board, most men need to drink about 101 fluid ounces (13 cups) a day, and most women should aim to drink about 74 fluid ounces (9 cups) a day. However, as your workouts get more intense in the weeks to come, and if you live in a hot climate, you may need to drink even more, depending on how much you sweat.

A good way to determine if you are drinking enough is to check your urine. Dark, scant urine generally indicates dehydration, while clear and frequent urine means you are on track. All those trips to the bathroom may seem inconvenient, but your body will thank you.

OPTIONS, OPTIONS You may be wondering how you will ever manage to guzzle that much water. Don't worry—you don't have to. Juices, milk, smoothies, sports drinks, and soft drinks all fulfill your fluid needs. Even drinks containing caffeine, like tea and coffee, and those containing alcohol count toward hydration. It is true that caffeine and alcohol are diuretics, as well, which means they force your body to eliminate water. But at the end of the day our bodies compensate for the water loss, so caffeinated and alcoholic beverages ultimately contribute to total water intake.

Water, though, is the best beverage. It is absorbed quickly and has no calories. Many studies have shown that water has an edge over other drinks when it comes

What's with All the Water?

It used to be simple—you just drank water from the tap. Then came bottled water. Now there's a plethora of enriched, enhanced, and flavored waters to choose from. Are any of them worth the money? And what's the best water for you?

First of all, many of us walk around dehydrated without realizing it, so simply making an effort to drink more water may make you feel better. It may help you shed pounds, too. One study found that women on a weight-loss program who drank more than 1 liter of water (about 4 cups) a day lost almost five pounds more over a year than those who drank less.

Sports drinks can be helpful for those training for an endurance event, like a marathon or triathlon, because they contain carbohydrates (sugars) and electrolytes (essential body salts) to replace some of what's lost during intense or prolonged exercise. But if you're an everyday exerciser, working out for less than an hour at a time, plain water will provide all the hydration your body needs—and zero calories. You can replace any lost electrolytes at your next meal.

In addition to sports drinks, some enhanced or "designer" waters contain vitamins and minerals; others contain substances ranging from caffeine to fiber to ginseng to natural flavorings. They may make a lot of health claims, but there's no proof that the designer waters are any better for you than the basic, ordinary kind. In fact, most are glorified soft drinks containing sugar or artificial sweeteners and, often, chemical food dyes.

I suggest you stick with good old water. Carry a bottle with you so that you are more likely to drink throughout the day. For the most economical and "green" option, invest in a good-quality reusable water bottle.

to the disease-prevention factors mentioned previously for cancers of the urinary tract and colon. That's why it is a good idea to get at least half of your daily fluid needs in the form of water. That rounds off to 5 cups of water a day for women and 7 cups of water a day for men, as a minimum.

CUT OUT THE SUGAR You can get the rest of your fluids from a number of different sources, as I mentioned. But clearly, all are not nutritionally equal. The most nutritious liquids are 100% juices, low-fat milk, soups, and healthy smoothies. One-hundred-percent juices are packed with nutrients like vitamin C, folic acid, and potassium. Low-fat milk provides calcium and essential B vitamins. And soups and smoothies are also loaded with vitamins and minerals. All of these foods have calories, of course, so keep portions in mind.

calories and added sugar in beverages

DRINK	CALORIES	ADDED SUGAR (TEASPOONS)*
Water	0	0
Latte, nonfat (8 oz.)	68	0
Milk, nonfat (8 oz.)	86	0
Beer, light (12 oz.)	100	0
Orange juice (8 oz.)	112	0
Latte, regular (8 oz.)	114	0
Wine (6 oz.)	124	0
Sweetened iced tea (12 oz.)	135–150	8–10
Soda (12 oz.)	145–150	10
Beer, regular (12 oz.)	147	0
Milk, whole (8 oz.)	150	0

*I have included added sugar as opposed to the naturally occurring sugars inherent in the food.

Sodas, soft drinks, sports drinks, enhanced waters, sweetened teas, and juice drinks are excellent hydrators, but they are loaded with calories and lack the nutrients of 100% juices and milk. They are basically sugar water, making it all too easy to suck up hundreds of empty calories through a straw.

Take Charles, for example, a 31-year-old investment banker from New York City, who came into my office completely perplexed. He was really pushing himself at the gym, he'd joined a basketball league, and he was eating very well—lots of vegetables, smaller portions, and no junk food. But despite all his efforts to trim down, he was gaining weight. He was very frustrated and about to give up.

Eventually I discovered Charles's problem: he was drinking almost a gallon of cranberry juice cocktail every day! He figured he needed fluids to rehydrate from his morning basketball game and thought he was making a healthy choice. He didn't realize that his "healthy" drink packed a whopping 1,000 calories! Charles didn't like plain water, so I suggested he try spiking his water with just a splash of the cranberry juice cocktail. Two weeks after making the switch, Charles came back, smiling, reporting a three-pound weight loss.

I have seen many cases like Charles. Most people don't realize how quickly they can drink their calories, and when they cut back on sugary drinks, they almost instantly lose weight. That makes sense when you stop to think that a 12-ounce can of soda has 150 calories and the equivalent of about 10 teaspoons of sugar. You can lose half a pound a week simply by cutting out two sodas a day! Talk about the benefits of small changes!

Diet drinks are an option if you want your soft drinks without the calories, but I do not recommend consuming artificial sweeteners. They train our tastebuds to be accustomed to intense sweetness, and although the FDA deems them safe, we never really know the effects of comsuming large quantities of them over time. For flavorful, low-cal options, try adding a splash of juice and/or a squeeze of lemon to ice water or club soda. Herbal teas, served hot or iced, are also a good hydrating choice, and many have a natural sweetness.

TEA Tea is the third most popular beverage in the United States, after water and coffee. It also appears to be one of the healthiest beverages you can drink.

Hundreds of published studies suggest that tea can inhibit or reduce your risk of a range of chronic diseases and conditions, from heart disease to bad breath. Tea contains powerful antioxidants called polyphenols, which have been shown to help protect your heart and guard against cancer. Tea also has an antimicrobial effect and may help reinforce the immune system. It has metabolism-boosting components that may aid in weight loss, as well.

Traditional tea—which includes black, oolong, green, and white tea—is derived from one plant, *Camellia sinensis*. When and how the tea leaves are harvested and the manner in which they are processed determines the strength and taste of the tea. Green tea and white tea are the least processed and are not fermented or oxidized, or broken and exposed to air for a period of time; as a result, they contain the most antioxidants. Oolong is partially oxidized, and black tea is fully oxidized. The exposure to air changes the color of the tea leaves (from green to black, for example) and the flavor of the tea. Black tea has the strongest taste, while white is the mildest, and all forms of tea contain caffeine (unless you choose a decaffeinated variety).

In addition to "true" tea, herbal teas (also called tisanes) provide their own healing effects. Herbal teas are made from herbs, flowers, and/or fruits but contain no actual tea, so they're naturally caffeine free. I use ginger tea to curb nausea and chamomile teas to aid in digestion. Medicinal properties aside, herbal teas are tasty quenchers with zero calories.

COFFEE Coffee used to get a bad rap as causing all kinds of health problems, but java lovers now have a lot to celebrate. It turns out that coffee is not only NOT bad for you but it has multiple health benefits! Studies over the past several years have shown that coffee reduces the risk of liver and rectal cancer, type 2 diabetes, Parkinson's disease, and gallstones. So now you can relax and enjoy your cup of joe without worry.

Still, when drinking tea and coffee, make sure to pay attention to fat and calories. Plain tea has just a calorie or so, but sweetened iced teas can have as much sugar and calories as soda. And a 16-ounce latte with whole milk tops off at 13 grams of fat and almost 250 calories—even before you add sugar to it!

COFFEE BREAK/TEA TIME The healing properties of tea and coffee are only part of their potential benefit. The simple act of relaxing with a warm cup of brew somehow immediately calms you down. Taking a special break for tea or coffee is a wonderful way to escape the stresses of the day. If you have the time and inclination, consider making a little ritual of it. Use a nice teapot or coffeepot and one of your favorite teacups or mugs. Break out the silverware and cloth napkins. Put on some soft music. Invite over a friend to chat, or just take some time for you. Sip slowly and enjoy. It is a healthy way to recharge and relax, all at the same time.

IS TOO MUCH JOE MAKING YOU JITTERY? Are you one of those people who can't function until your first cup of coffee? Are you hooked on a midmorning latte, or do you rely on diet sodas to keep you going through a long afternoon? While caffeine is the most widely used drug in the world, it can have some negative health consequences you should be aware of.

Caffeine boosts alertness, and research has found that it can help ease headaches (that's the reason it's found in some pain relievers). It's also been shown to boost physical performance when taken before exercise. That's the good news.

The bad news is that as a stimulant, it may raise your blood pressure, and too much can make you jittery. It also has a natural laxative effect (which can be good or bad, depending) and can cause heartburn and worsen ulcer pain.

What does this mean for you? As with most things, moderation is the safest bet. People's tolerance levels vary—you may be able to drink three cups of coffee with no ill effects, while your friend is wired after a can of cola. But in general, it's a good idea to keep your caffeine consumption under 300 milligrams a day. (Refer to the Caffeine Content of Some Popular Beverages chart on page 104 to help you calculate.)

One note: if you decide to cut back on your intake, do it gradually to avoid possible headaches from going "cold turkey." If you're looking for caffeine-free beverages, drink herbal teas and decaf coffee, and check the labels on your soft drinks. Many non-cola beverages contain caffeine.

caffeine content of some popular beverages

DRINK	CAFFEINE
Coffee, brewed (8 oz.)	100–200 mg
Latte (16 oz.)	150–170 mg
Instant coffee (8 oz.)	60–85 mg
Black tea (8 oz.)	25–50 mg
Soda (12 oz.)	35–70 mg
Iced tea (12 oz.)	15–75 mg

ALCOHOL A lot of people jumped for joy when they heard the reports that alcohol has a protective effect on the heart. "Finally something seemingly sinful is good for me!" they cheered. In fact, a moderate amount of alcohol can be good for your heart health. Research shows that drinking any type of alcohol in moderation can lower your risk of stroke, raise good cholesterol (HDL), and lower bad cholesterol (LDL). Red wine produces these positive effects, and more. It contains a type of antioxidant called resveratrol that can further protect the heart.

That's all great news. But hold on, because once you drink past the point of moderation (which is defined as one drink a day for women and two for men), alcohol's benefits are quickly swallowed up by the risks. Heavy drinking can really take a toll, leading to liver disease, stroke, cancer, and many other ailments. Alcohol also has plenty of calories. So if you don't drink, don't start. But if you do, enjoy. Just take it easy.

action

Your action this week is to get enough total fluids every day, and make sure at least half of your fluid intake is water. For most people that means between 72 and 104 fluid ounces (nine to thirteen 8-ounce glasses of liquid total), including *at least* five to seven glasses of water. Also, cut your intake of soda and sugary soft drinks to no more than one a day.

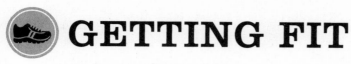

GETTING FIT

strength training

At this point, you've been walking three times a week and now are adding stretching after your walks. Believe it or not, you're already a quarter of the way through the program.

The next step is strength training. Even if you've never lifted a weight in your life, strength-building moves are an essential component of any fitness regimen. That doesn't mean you have to join a gym and start pumping iron—some of the most effective moves are ones you can do anytime, anyplace.

The objective of this week is to introduce the idea of strength training and to show you how easy it is to incorporate some into your fitness plan.

WHY STRENGTH TRAINING? Cardiovascular exercises such as walking, biking, and swimming are great for strengthening your heart, burning calories, and reducing stress. But they go only so far to help you build and maintain muscle mass.

You likely don't want huge, bulging muscles. But if you want a sleek, toned look—and a stronger, more injury-proof body—then strength training is for you. More than that, it should be an essential part of everyone's exercise routine: the American College of Sports Medicine recommends that adults perform at least one set of strengthening moves at least two or three times a week.

Does strength training bring to mind sweaty guys pumping iron in a gym? Simply put, strength training (also called resistance training or weight training) involves challenging a muscle (or group of muscles) beyond what it normally does. You do this using your body weight, free weights or dumbbells, exercise machines, exercise bands, or other equipment to provide resistance for the muscle to work against.

That effort creates microscopic tears in the muscle that are rebuilt by your body over the next couple of days. The result is denser, stronger, and sometimes—depending on how you train—bigger muscle. (You need not worry about bulking up—professional bodybuilders train daily and intensively to achieve their eye-popping physiques.)

Not yet convinced? Well, strength training offers numerous benefits for both women and men:

- **It improves your appearance.** Cardiovascular exercise is great for reducing stress and burning calories, but it won't change the basic shape of your body. Nothing sculpts your body like resistance training—you must overload your muscles beyond what they normally do to tone them up. And firm muscles also help mask the appearance of cellulite by smoothing out lumps of fat underneath the skin.

- **It boosts your metabolism.** Strength training helps make your body a more efficient fat-burning machine. Every pound of muscle you gain burns about 50 calories a day, even at rest, meaning that when you have more muscle, you can eat more and maintain your weight—or that you'll lose weight without changing your caloric intake. Because muscle weighs more than fat, you may not see the scale move as you build muscle and lose fat, but you'll notice that you look slimmer and leaner and your clothes fit better.

- **It keeps you young.** As you age, you begin to lose muscle and bone mass, but strength training can stave off those losses. Strength training helps maintain bone mass to combat osteoporosis. Strong bones also help you maintain good posture and make you less likely to suffer a fracture as you age.

- **It makes you tougher.** Not only do you look better, you're less injury prone—the stronger your muscles are, the less likely you are to get hurt. (It is important to start off slowly with any strength-training program, as we are doing this week, to make sure you're not overdoing it at first.)

- **It reduces anxiety.** Studies show that strength training reduces anxiety and eases depression. At the end of a particularly crazy day, you may find that performing some strengthening moves helps you work off your tension. You're forced to concentrate on what you're doing instead of what's bothering you.

- **It improves your posture.** Those strong bones and muscles mean you'll walk taller. And not only will you stand straighter, you'll feel more confident, as well—research shows that weight lifting improves self-esteem.

- **It makes life easier.** Because strength training—obviously—makes you stronger, you're better able to perform functional tasks like carrying groceries or picking up your two-year-old. That makes you more efficient in your daily life, too.

Besides keeping you strong and healthy, strength training can radically improve your appearance. Many people focus on cardiovascular exercise, neglecting resistance training. Thirty-seven-year-old Cindy, a human resources professional, had been a treadmill junkie. She walked religiously but didn't notice a difference in her body until she began strength training. She started lifting weights, exercising in the mornings before she went to work, and was pleasantly surprised by the results.

Within three months, Cindy could see a noticeable improvement in her overall physique. "I weigh the same, but I've lost inches," she said. "I'm firmer and more toned. It's not like I've suddenly got huge muscles, either—it's just changed the shape of my body." Her arms and legs are slimmer, and now when she shops for clothes, she looks for sleeveless tops and shorts to show off her now defined, sleek muscles.

Tracking Your Progress

You've been using your Food and Exercise Journal to track your workouts, but if you prefer a higher-tech approach, check out these websites that are all free to join. You can measure your progress, tally your calories, and connect with like-minded people:

- **www.fitday**
  This site includes an online diet journal and detailed nutrition information for thousands of foods.

- **www.mynetdiary**
  Here you can track the amount of calories you eat in a day.

- **www.onlinefitnesslog**
  Allows you to track, plan, and personalize your exercise plan.

SMART ADVICE ABOUT DUMBBELLS While you can use a variety of equipment for strength building, you may want to buy dumbbells to have at home. They're inexpensive and designed to be easy to grip. (Look for versions that are padded to protect your hands.)

Visit a sporting goods store and experiment to determine which weight is right for you. (Start off with a light weight—maybe two or five pounds—so you won't hurt yourself!) Choose a weight that you can do 10 to 12 repetitions with before you're tired; you may want to get several sets of dumbbells so that you can use them for different moves. Typically you'll use a heavier weight for lower body, lighter weights for upper body.

Another option is to purchase exercise bands. They're even cheaper than dumbbells, smaller, lighter, and easy to store or pack. Exercise bands come in different colors and resistances; a home set will cost you about $15.

SEVEN SUPER STRENGTHENERS While some people work out with free weights (barbells and dumbbells), and others use weight machines at the gym, you don't need expensive equipment to get started. Some of the most effective moves—like push-ups and crunches—simply use your body's weight as resistance instead of a machine.

These seven simple moves target your major muscle groups and will strengthen and tone you. Add them to your walking routine, after you walk and before you stretch. For a couple of these exercises, you'll need a dumbbell or an exercise band. But if you don't want to buy any equipment, take a look in your pantry: you can use a 16-ounce can, or put several cans in a plastic grocery bag.

Start with one set of 8 to 12 reps of each exercise, and concentrate on doing each move slowly—you'll get more results.

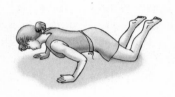

Modified push-ups (targets chest and triceps, the muscles along the backs of your arms) With your body facing down toward the floor and your knees slightly bent, hands at your shoulders, support your weight on your hands and knees. Keeping your body straight, lower yourself to a few inches off the ground and press back up. (If you're in good shape already, you can start off with your weight on your hands and toes, which makes it more difficult.) Do 8 to 12 reps.

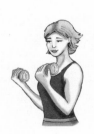

Biceps curls (targets the muscles along the fronts of your arms) Stand with feet shoulder width apart, dumbbells (or cans or other weights) in both hands, or holding the handles of an exercise band in your hands. With your arms at your sides, bend your elbows and bring your hands up toward your shoulders, keeping your elbows in and slightly in front against your body and your shoulders back, then slowly lower them back down. Do 8 to 12 reps.

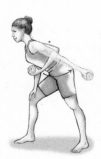

Triceps kickbacks (targets the backs of your arms) Stand and step forward with your right foot so that it's about two feet in front of you. Hold a dumbbell, can, or the handle of an exercise band in your left hand with your arm bent, lean forward, and place your right hand on your right knee for support. Keeping your left upper arm tucked against your body, straighten your arm and then return to your original position. Do 8 to 12 reps, and then switch sides and repeat with your left leg forward and working your right arm.

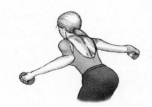

Back flys (targets the muscles of your back) Bend forward at the hips, keeping your legs straight and knees relaxed, and hold a dumbbell, can, or exercise strap handle in each hand. Keeping your body stable and your palms facing in, lift your elbows up and bring your arms up and away from your body, until your elbows are level with your shoulders; then return to your original position. Do 8 to 12 reps.

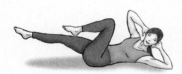

Bicycles (targets abdominal muscles) Lie on your back, legs lifted off the floor, knees slightly bent, hands behind your head. Straighten and lower your legs toward the floor one at a time; as you do so, lift your head and shoulders off the ground and twist your right shoulder toward your left knee as the right leg lowers toward the floor and vice versa. Be careful not to bring in your elbows and pull your neck, just cradle it with your hands. Do 8 to 12 reps.

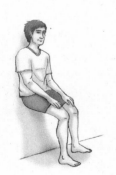

Wall squats (targets the muscles in your legs and your butt) Stand with your feet slightly wider than hip width, about 12 to 18 inches from a wall, your back against the wall, legs slightly bent. Slowly slide your back down the wall, bending your legs as if you were going to sit down. Keep your weight on your heels and lower your body to a few inches above a full sitting position. Make sure your feet are far enough out so that your shins are perpendicular to the floor. Hold here for 3 to 5 full breaths. Return to your original position. Repeat 3 times.

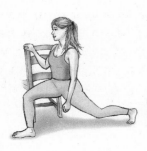

Lunges (targets the legs and butt) Stand straight next to a sturdy chair, with your feet shoulder width apart. Holding the chair for balance, step forward with your right foot, making a large enough step so that your shin stays perpendicular to the ground when you lower your body; push back up and return to your original position. Do 8 to 12 reps.

action

Perform these strengthening moves three times this week in addition to doing your 20-minute walks and stretching. You may find it easiest to add the strength moves at the end of your walk, but feel free to do them at a different time of day (or even a different day) if you prefer. Just make sure you give yourself a day off in between the strengthening moves, to let your muscles recover.

 # FEELING GOOD

better sleep

I can't tell you how many times people have asked me what kinds of foods they can eat for more energy or to improve the way they feel. When I chat with them further, I discover that they're sleeping no more than five or six hours a night (or less)—no wonder they feel tired! You can eat more healthfully, get more exercise, and reduce your stress levels, but if you're not sleeping enough, you're still not going to feel great. Simply sleeping more is often overlooked as a life-enhancing technique, yet sleep is essential for good health and a positive frame of mind.

Researchers don't know exactly *why* sleep is so critical to good health, but we do know that during sleep, a variety of essential functions occur, including repair, growth, and maintenance of the body's tissues, regulating immune function, and suppressing the production of stress hormones.

Lack of sleep causes problems in many areas. First is a safety issue—people who don't get enough sleep are more likely to fall asleep while driving or get injured on the job. Then there's how lack of sleep affects day-to-day life. When people don't get enough sleep, they're often tired, moody, or irritable, which affects their relationships at home and at work. Lack of sleep also has an impact on our ability to concentrate, think, and carry out even mundane tasks; it's also linked to depression and anxiety. Inadequate sleep is linked to cardiovascular disease such as heart attacks and strokes, as well as to impaired immune system function. New studies also suggest it makes you more likely to gain weight and may make it harder to control diabetes.

The 2010 Sleep in America poll conducted by the National Sleep Foundation found that only about 40% of Americans are getting adequate sleep most nights—and that means 60% of us aren't sleeping well the majority of the time. And while sleep needs vary, 30% of us get fewer than six hours of sleep/night, far short of what most people need for overall health and productivity.

Power Napping

In some cultures, it's the norm to take a midafternoon siesta. That's when most people's energy levels dip. A short nap at this time can refresh and energize you for the rest of the day. A few tips on daytime snoozing:

- **Make yourself comfortable.** That may mean stretching out on your couch or bed at home, or putting your head down on your desk at work.

- **Make your area quiet.** Earplugs can help drown out office chatter, or you can shut the door if you have one.

- **Set an alarm.** You won't enjoy your siesta if you're worried you're going to oversleep.

- **Limit your sleep time.** A short nap—about 15 minutes—appears to be optimal, according to research. If you nap longer than that, you may feel groggy or find it harder to fall asleep later that night.

- **Run it by your boss.** You don't want to be caught napping on the job without clearing it with your supervisor first. Mention that you're going to cut your lunch break short and use the time to take a short nap later to help boost your productivity. How can he or she say no to that?

HOW MUCH SLEEP DO YOU NEED? Researchers agree that the optimum amount of sleep for each person varies. Some people thrive on five or six hours of sleep, while others feel better with eight or even nine hours. Babies, children, and teenagers need more sleep than adults. The amount of physical activity you perform can also affect the amount you need—you may need more rest after a strenuous day, for example.

You may already know how much sleep you need by assessing how you feel after sleeping different amounts. If you feel well rested after seven hours each night, that's probably your optimum amount. If you need eight and a half to feel human in the morning, shoot for that.

Though most of us occasionally have to sacrifice sleep, remember that it will catch up with you. Sure, there will be times when you're unable to sleep or are up with a sick child or simply can't get your mind to stop racing. By making sleep a priority, you'll set yourself up for a more restful slumber.

Getting enough sleep does more than make you more clear-headed the next day. It may also make it easier to shed pounds and maintain your weight. If you've ever found yourself reaching for a cinnamon roll or candy bar in an attempt to energize after a sleepless night, it will come as no surprise that people who don't sleep well are hungrier than those who do.

A recent study found that people who had their sleep restricted for several nights had more food cravings and consumed more food overall than those who slept normally. Other research has linked short sleep duration and weight gain, and it now appears that women who sleep the fewest number of hours are the most likely to become obese. The cause may be in part due to the fact that lack of sleep causes hormone alterations that not only make you feel hungry but affect your metabolism, making you more likely to gain weight.

SLEEPING BETTER It's not simply how many hours of sleep you get—it's the quality, as well. If you constantly wake up during the night, you won't feel as rested in the morning.

Less-than-stellar-quality sleep is a common complaint—7 in 10 people say they experience frequent sleep problems. Yet there are many ways to improve your sleep:

- **Set a regular schedule.** Try to go to bed and get up at the same time each day. This will help set your "body clock."

- **Create a wind-down routine for yourself.** If you've parented young children, you've probably done this with them to get ready for bed—first they put on their pajamas, then they brush their teeth, then it's time for a story. Create your own bedtime routine. That might mean taking a warm bath or curling up with a favorite book for a few minutes. Allow yourself time to wind down before you get in bed, and you're more likely to sleep better.

- **Cut back on TV.** The vast majority of us spend the last hour before bed watching TV several nights a week. If you're watching something educational or fun, a little TV before bed might be relaxing. However, catching up on financial news or watching a violent drama may make you more prone to tossing and turning.

- **Unplug.** If you use your bed as a second office, stop—and take your laptop out of your bedroom. Your bed should be a respite from the world and should be used only for sleep and sex. Put away your smartphone, laptop, and other electronics to prepare for a restful night. It's a good idea to keep the TV out of the bedroom, too.

- **Create a restful environment.** Your bedroom should be dark, quiet, and a comfortable temperature—neither too hot nor too cold.

- **Go easy on the alcohol.** Alcohol makes you sleepy at first, but it reduces the quality and depth of sleep and can ultimately lead to a restless night.

- **Raise your body temperature—to drop it.** There's some truth to a warm bath helping produce restful sleep—your body temperature drops after the bath, which makes you feel relaxed and sleepy.

- **Exercise gently.** If you work out a few hours before bed, it will probably affect your sleep quality because your metabolism is still running high. Some light stretching or yoga poses are fine before bed, but higher-intensity workouts should come earlier in the day.

- **Eat lightly.** A heavy meal late at night is likely to affect your sleep because your body's busy digesting it. A light snack is fine—milk or a carbohydrate-rich snack like whole-grain crackers or a piece of fruit could help relax you.

action

This week, create a bedtime ritual for yourself. It need not be anything extravagant—just come up with a routine that will tell your body it's time to get ready for sleep. It might be washing your face and brushing your teeth before you climb into bed, or taking a few minutes to read before you slip under the covers. Set your alarm (if you use one) for the same time every morning, and try to get to bed around the same time, as well—you'll sleep better in the long run.

week 4 ACTION SUMMARY

eating well

- Shop to replenish your healthy pantry.
- Stay between 3 and 7 on the Hunger Continuum (see page 61).
- Eat three meals and one or two snacks each day.
- Drink at least five glasses of water and no more than one soda or other sugary beverage each day.
- Maintain your food journal.

getting fit

- Walk for 20 minutes at low to mid-intensity three times.
- Stretch and do strength training three times.
- Note your exercise activities in your journal.

feeling good

- Do the Five-Minute Breathing Exercise daily.
- Practice mindfulness.
- Say no to tasks you don't want to and don't have to do.
- Create a bedtime ritual.

WEIGHT

....

WEEK 5

this week's changes

1. Get enough healthy fat each day, and skip the bad fat.

2. Do something active just for fun!

3. Incorporate a minivacation or play break into your day.

this week's recipes

De"light"ful Dressings, Dips, Spreads, and Sauces

- Citrus-Ginger Dressing
- Balsamic Vinaigrette
- Mustard-Dill Sauce
- Creamy Honey Walnut Spread
- Roasted Garlic
- Roasted Tomato Sauce

Fat does make food taste good, and you can have both taste and health if you choose the right fats in the right amounts. These luscious recipes are proof, so drizzle, dip, and spread away!

citrus-ginger dressing

SERVES 6 *This dressing has a bright, slightly sweet, and tangy flavor. Try it on a green salad garnished with sliced almonds and orange sections or maybe some thinly sliced fennel. Use it also for Citrus-Ginger Flounder with Snow Peas on page 209.*

¼ cup orange juice

3 tablespoons lemon juice

1 tablespoon white wine vinegar

2 tablespoons canola oil

1 tablespoon honey

1 tablespoon peeled and freshly grated ginger

Salt and freshly ground black pepper to taste

In a small bowl, whisk together all the ingredients until well blended.

Calories 59; Fat 4.6 g (Sat .3 g, Mono 2.7 g, Poly 1.3 g); Protein .1 g; Carb 4.8 g; Fiber .1 g; Chol 0 mg; Sodium .6 mg

balsamic vinaigrette

SERVES 6 *This vinaigrette is made lighter with the addition of chicken or vegetable broth, which takes the place of about half the oil used in a typical recipe. It turns out much lower in calories but equally flavorful.*

¼ cup balsamic vinegar
¼ cup extra-virgin olive oil
¼ cup low-sodium chicken or vegetable broth
1 tablespoon Dijon mustard
Salt and freshly ground black pepper to taste

In a small bowl, whisk together all of the ingredients until well blended.

Calories 90; Fat 9 g (Sat 1.3 g, Mono 6.6 g, Poly .8 g); Protein 2 g; Carb 1.4 g; Fiber 0 g; Chol .2 mg; Sodium 63 mg

mustard-dill sauce

SERVES 4 *Yogurt is my go-to ingredient for making creamy rich sauces and dips with a fraction of the calories and little or no mayonnaise. This sauce is delicious for dipping raw vegetables. Also use it on Poached Salmon with Mustard-Dill Sauce (page 210).*

½ cup low-fat plain yogurt
2 teaspoons Dijon mustard
2 teaspoons lemon juice
1 tablespoon chopped fresh dill

In a small bowl, whisk together all the ingredients until well blended.

Calories 20; Fat 0 g; Protein 1.8 g; Carb 2.6 g; Fiber 0 g; Chol 6 mg; Sodium 81 mg

creamy honey walnut spread

SERVES 4 *Use this satisfying spread instead of cream cheese or butter on toast or a bagel. Top with sliced fruit for a tasty, colorful nutrition boost.*

⅓ cup shelled walnuts
⅔ cup nonfat plain Greek-style yogurt
2 teaspoons honey

1. Preheat the oven to 400°F. Spread the walnuts on a baking sheet and toast in the oven for about 5 minutes. Be careful not to let them burn. When they have cooled, chop them very fine.

2. Put the yogurt in a small bowl. Stir in the walnuts and honey, and serve.

Calories 90; Fat 5 g (Sat .5 g, Mono .7 g, Poly 3.9 g); Protein 5 g; Carb 6 g; Fiber 1 g; Chol 0 mg; Sodium 15 mg

roasted garlic

SERVES 4 TO 6 *Roasted garlic is one of the most versatile and delicious flavorings around. The roasting mellows the garlic and brings out a rich sweetness. I like to serve it as a bread-spread instead of butter or use it on sandwiches.*

2 heads of garlic
1 tablespoon olive oil
  Salt to taste

1. Preheat the oven to 375°F. Remove the outermost papery skin from the garlic and cut off the top quarter of the head so that the cloves are exposed. Put the garlic, cut side up, into a small roasting pan, drizzle with the olive oil, and cover the pan with foil. Bake in the oven for about 1 hour, until the garlic is soft and golden brown.

2. Serve the garlic head whole so that guests can scoop the soft garlic out of each clove themselves with a knife and spread it on bread. Or squeeze the garlic out before serving it, puree it with a little more olive oil, and serve as a spread. Season with salt to taste.

Calories 52; Fat 3.4 g (Sat .5 g, Mono 2.5 g, Poly .3 g); Protein .9 g; Carb 5 g; Fiber .3 g; Chol 0 mg; Sodium 2.5 mg

roasted tomato sauce

SERVES 4 *You can make this easy tomato sauce any time of year, but it is best in the summer when the tomatoes are in peak season and at their most flavorful. A little orange juice is the secret ingredient to punch up the tomatoes' natural sweetness. It just requires a touch of healthy oil, so it is very low in calories.*

   Cooking spray
2 pints (1¼ pounds) grape tomatoes, halved (4½ cups)
4 garlic cloves, halved, plus 1 clove, minced
1 tablespoon olive oil
1 medium onion, chopped (1¼ cups)
2 tablespoons tomato paste
1 tablespoon orange juice
2 tablespoons chopped fresh basil
   Salt and freshly ground black pepper to taste

1. Preheat the broiler and lightly spray a foil-lined baking sheet with oil. Put the tomatoes on a baking sheet and distribute the halved garlic evenly among the tomatoes. Place under the broiler for about 5 minutes, checking occasionally to stir, until the tomatoes are slightly charred.

2. Heat the olive oil in a heavy saucepan over moderate heat and cook the onion until softened, about 3 minutes. Add the roasted tomatoes and the tomato paste and cook, stirring, for 5 minutes.

3. Transfer the mixture to a blender and puree with the orange juice. Stir in the basil. Season with salt and pepper to taste.

Calories 80; Fat 4 g (Sat .5 g, Mono 2.5 g, Poly .5 g) ; Protein 2 g; Carb 11 g; Fiber 3 g; Chol 0 mg; Sodium 75 mg

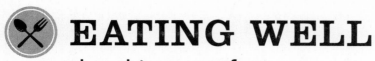

EATING WELL
the skinny on fat

"Eat less fat," "Stick to the right kinds of fat," "Don't cut out too much fat." It seems like advice about fat—how much and what kind to eat—flip-flops with the seasons, leaving many people understandably confused and frustrated. This week, I'm going to clear up the confusion and show you how fat not only fits into a healthy and satisfying way of eating but in fact is an essential component of it.

IS FAT BAD? In the 1980s, the major message coming from many nutrition experts was that fat is bad, and the less fat you eat, the better. The reasoning went that fat contributes to heart disease by increasing blood cholesterol. It also promotes weight gain, since it packs more than twice the calories per gram (9 calories a gram) as carbohydrates or proteins, which each have 4 calories a gram. Experts declared that fat is a big culprit in making America obese.

At the time, it seemed to make sense—eat fat, get fat. But our knowledge about fats has evolved in the past decades. We now know that simply reducing our fat intake won't necessarily make us thin or healthy. In fact, it turns out that when we replace fats with sugars, it can be even worse for our health! Americans, as a population, have managed to gain even more weight after switching to sugary low-fat cookies and fat-free ice cream. And we have discovered that while some kinds of fat are harmful, others are beneficial to your health and should be encouraged.

Fat is an essential part of your diet. It makes food taste better and can provide additional calories to those who need them. Your body needs fat to absorb fat-soluble vitamins, and it's essential for healthy skin, hair, and cells. It also has some other important health benefits.

GOOD FATS Not all fats are created equal. There are two main types of fats: saturated, which are solid at room temperature; and unsaturated, which are liquid at room temperature. As a general rule, the unsaturated fats are the healthy fats you want to be eating. Replacing saturated fats—primarily those that come from animal products like meat, cheese, and eggs—with unsaturated fats can lower your cholesterol, protect your heart, and prevent other diseases.

Unsaturated fats are grouped into two categories—monounsaturated and polyunsaturated, each with its own positive qualities. Olive oil, olives, canola oil, peanut oil, avocados, cashews, and almonds are all foods rich in monounsaturated fat. This type of fat helps lowers bad cholesterol (LDL) while maintaining good cholesterol (HDL) and has been shown to protect against heart disease, stroke, and cancer.

Polyunsaturated fats come in two types—omega-3 and omega-6. Both are essential—you must obtain them from your diet to prevent a deficiency. Omega-3 and omega-6 fats are both critical to the health of all of our cells, especially those associated with the skin and the immune system, but they play different roles in our bodies.

Omega-3 fat lowers bad cholesterol while keeping good cholesterol stable, and it helps reduce tissue inflammation, which is thought to be at the root of heart disease, stroke, and arthritis. Reams of evidence point to omega-3 as the healthiest fat, yet most of us do not get enough of it. The best sources of omega-3 fat are fish, especially fatty fish like salmon, sardines, and tuna. You can also get omega-3 from vegetable sources like flaxseed, walnuts, and green leafy vegetables, but the type of omega-3 in these foods is not as potent as that found in fish.

Omega-6 fat is a mixed bag. It is essential, and it lowers cholesterol when eaten in place of saturated fat. But it lowers both bad cholesterol *and* good cholesterol, and has been linked with an increase in the inflammation that contributes to disease. Some big omega-6 sources include soybean oil, sunflower oil, corn oil, and mayonnaise made with these oils. Many foods, like walnuts, tofu, and wheat germ are rich in both omega-3 and omega-6 fats.

Eating a mixture of the three types of unsaturated fats—mono, omega-3, and omega-6—is important. Most of us get more than enough omega-6 fat from salad dressings and cooking oils, especially when dining out. The key to consuming more healthful fats is getting more omega-3 and monounsaturated fats into your diet.

That means eating more fish, nuts, avocado, and tofu, including wheat germ and ground flaxseed in your favorite foods (sprinkle them on yogurt or cereal, or put them in muffin and pancake batter), and using olive oil, canola oil, peanut oil, and flaxseed oil and nut oils. Keep in mind that flaxseed oil and nut oil are very sensitive to light and heat, so you should not cook with them. Use them in salad dressings or drizzle on cooked foods instead.

BAD FATS Now you know the basics about the good fats. There are two kinds of fat that should be limited—saturated fats and trans fats. As I mentioned earlier, saturated fat is solid at room temperature and is found in foods like meat, full-fat milk and yogurt, cheese, cream, and butter. It is also the primary fat in tropical fruit oils like coconut and palm oil (see The Coconut Oil Controversy on page 124). Saturated fat raises bad cholesterol, which is a risk factor for heart disease. While you don't need to eliminate saturated fat altogether, it should be limited to less than 10% of your total calories.

Trans fat is one fat you should try to cut out completely. It is worse for your heart than saturated fat, because it raises bad cholesterol *and* lowers good cholesterol. Trans fat is formed when oil is hydrogenated, or processed to become solid. It is found in stick margarine, vegetable shortening, fried foods, and most commercially packaged baked goods, crackers, pastries, cookies, and other products.

Since 2006, food producers have had to specifically list grams of trans fats on food labels; before that, you had to look for the words *hydrogenated* or *partially hydrogenated vegetable oil* on the ingredient list. Due to both the new labeling requirements and to consumer pressure, many food manufacturers have reformulated products to limit or eliminate trans fats, so the problem is not as pervasive as it used to be. But you can still find plenty of trans fats in packaged and restaurant foods. Keep in mind that even if a food label says "zero trans fats," it can legally have up to .5 g per serving. If you eat a few servings, you could be unwittingly consuming a significant amount of trans fat.

Luckily, you don't need to remember all the details to get a good balance of the right kinds of fats. Simply sticking to the Usually/Sometimes/Rarely food lists (pages 14–16) will ensure that. There I've designated the healthiest fats as Usually or Sometimes foods, and the not-so-healthy fats as Rarely.

HOW MUCH FAT? When it comes to health, it seems that the kind of fat we eat is more important than the amount. But healthy or not, all fats have the same number of calories, and those calories can add up quickly. So if you are watching your waistline, dipping your bread in a dish of olive oil may be healthy for your heart, but it won't necessarily help you stay trim. You don't need to walk around counting fat grams all day long, but having an idea of how much fat you should be eating each day and becoming aware of the sources of fat in your diet can help you make better food decisions that ultimately help you lose weight.

I recommend eating a diet that contains a moderate amount of fat—about 30% of your total calories. To figure out how much fat you need, first determine your calorie range from the chart in Appendix A, How Much Should You Eat?, on page 291. Make a note of the calorie range you fall into, because you will use that as your guide for the rest of the Eating Well changes in this book.

If you are in group I, you should aim for 40 to 50 grams of fat per day; group II, 50 to 60 grams; group III, 60 to 70 grams; group IV, 70 to 85 grams; and group V, 85 to 100 grams of fat each day. If you keep that number of fat grams in mind as your "ceiling," next time you check the label on a box of doughnuts, you might be inspired to skip it. Besides passing on the doughnuts, simple changes like switching to low-fat milk, yogurt, and cheeses, choosing extra-lean meats, and opting for low-fat baked goods can help you keep your fat intake in check. Get the fat you need from healthy food sources like nuts, fish, avocado, and tofu.

These are all changes we will make in the weeks to come, so while you may incorporate them if you'd like, don't worry about them yet. This week's change focuses on added fat—the fat you put in or on food to make it taste better, as in dressings and spreads, and the fat that you cook with.

The chart below gives you an idea of how much fat is in different foods.

how much fat is in that?

FOOD	AMOUNT	FAT (G)
Low-fat milk, 1%	1 cup	2
Chocolate chip cookie	1 small	4
Egg	1 whole	5
Tofu	½ cup	5
Salad dressing, regular	1 tablespoon	6
Avocado	¼ avocado	8
Butter	2 teaspoons	8
Whole milk	1 cup	8
Cheddar cheese	1 ounce	9
Oil (all types)	2 teaspoons	9
Cream cheese	2 tablespoons	10
Salmon	4 ounces	13
Peanut butter	2 tablespoons	16
Ground beef, 85% lean	4 ounces	17
Nuts	¼ cup	18

THE COCONUT OIL CONTROVERSY Coconut oil has long been on the list of fats to avoid, because although it is from a fruit, it contains primarily saturated fat. But over the past few years, coconut oil has been touted as a wonder food, credited with improving immune function, aiding weight loss, and reducing the risk of heart disease, cancer, and many other ailments. Advocates argue that coconut oil is easier to absorb and is processed differently than other saturated fats because it consists mostly of medium-chain fatty acids, as opposed to the long-chain fatty acids found in animal fats.

It may not be as bad for us as once thought, but there isn't enough research to substantiate most of the health claims, and the main type of saturated fat it contains does significantly increase cholesterol. Until the verdict is in, I suggest keeping it on the Rarely list and focusing on monounsaturated and omega-3-rich oils.

Bread Spreads

For me, nothing beats the flavor of butter on toast in the morning. But because butter is so full of saturated fat, I use healthier, but still delicious, spreads most of the time and save the butter as a special treat. Some of my favorite toast toppers are peanut butter or almond butter and jam or honey, a smear of ripe avocado and a slice of tomato, or even a drizzle of olive oil and a little salt. I also love my Creamy Honey Walnut Spread (page 118).

action

Get two to four servings (depending on your calorie range) of healthy fats each day by cooking with them or using them on food. Reduce your intake of trans and saturated fats.

GETTING FIT

adding fun to fitness

This week, I want to talk about the importance of play in both your workout routine and your life in general.

FUN + FITNESS = RESULTS Think about the reasons you exercise. It may be to reduce stress, protect your health, or lose weight—or a combination of all three. But in search of achieving results, you may be forgetting that fitness can be fun.

If you're skeptical, bear with me. Physical activity can be enjoyable—you may have discovered by now that you like the feeling of walking or look forward to your thrice-weekly workouts as time for yourself. You may have found that even if you start your walk reluctantly, once you get going, you feel alive and invigorated. When you like what you're doing, you'll reap even more benefits—you're more likely to stick with your exercise program and you'll push yourself harder because you're more caught up in what you're doing. That means more results from your program.

As a child, Monica dreaded phys ed. She wasn't a particularly coordinated kid, and the calisthenics her gym teachers put her through turned her off to exercise for good. She envisioned the gym as a place where people suffered, and she had no interest in fitness classes of any kind. That changed when one of her friends dragged her to a Zumba class.

"I couldn't believe how fun it was!" says Monica. "The music was great, and I loved the camaraderie of the class. We were dancing and laughing and having a blast." Now she's a Zumba convert and takes a class three times a week.

"I was sore the next day, but I was having so much fun I didn't even realize I was exercising," she says. "I actually love working out now."

Fun exercise (come on, it's not an oxymoron!) can also help change your mindset that working out has to be a difficult or boring chore. To get in touch with the joy of movement, watch young children at play. They're not worrying about burning calories or building strong bones or staying flexible. They're not putting in their required exercise time so that they can check it off their mental list or log it in their journal. No, they're completely absorbed in what they're doing, whether they're zooming around as airplanes, jumping rope, or playing in a sandbox where they create cities of their own.

That rapt attention is what makes play so beneficial for children and adults both—during play, you can enter a state of flow where you're so focused on what you're doing that you forget everything else. In fact, flow is similar to a meditative state; the difference is that when you're performing an activity—playing the piano, practicing your tennis serve, or writing a novel—you're completely absorbed in the process.

ADDING FUN TO THE MIX What does this mean for you? It means that the more you enjoy exercise, the less painful it feels, and the more likely you are to stick with it. After a few weeks, most people find that exercising becomes its own reward—they feel so much better afterward that it motivates them to keep up their routine. But if activity still feels like a chore, here are a few ways to inject some fun into your regimen:

- **Shift your exercise time.** If you usually sleep as late as possible before crawling out of bed, get up early and walk first thing in the morning. If you usually exercise in the morning, opt for a lunch-hour or early-evening workout instead. Simply changing the setting or the time of day you exercise can make a big difference in your attitude.

what's fresh in fitness?

Walking may be the exercise mainstay (it's the easiest for most of us, after all), but if you find yourself getting bored already, mix up your routine with a new activity. Fitness trends come and go, but trying a new class can be a fun challenge for you. Check your local health club, Y, or community center to see what's offered. Some of the most popular classes today include the following (you'll find more exercise class options in Week 8 on page 199):

- **Body pump.** This weight-training class has been popular for years. If you want the benefits of pumping iron but are put off by the idea of hitting the weight room, this is a great option. You lift weights as a group, to music, and can choose dumbbells as light or as heavy as you like.

- **Boot camp.** Don't be put off by the name. Boot camp classes are great options if you want a serious workout without having to plan it; the instructor puts the group through challenging, body-weight-focused calisthenics and moves.

- **Kettle bells.** These shaped dumbbells have become increasingly popular. Research shows that kettle-bell workouts burn lots of calories, and they are a fun way to strength-train.

- **NIA.** The acronym stands for neuromuscular integrative action, but don't let the medical-sounding name put you off. This unique blend of modern dance, yoga, tai chi, and martial arts is low-impact but can be as intense as you want to make it.

- **Suspension training**. One of the newest classes out there (though not a completely new idea), suspension training uses strong, stretchy bands and webbing that attach to a stationary, stable object (like the ceiling or a pole) and let you work your muscles in different planes of motion. You use your body weight and gravity to develop strength, flexibility, and balance.

- **Yogalates or PiYo.** This class combines yoga and Pilates to give you some of the benefits of each. It's often less intense than a full-length Pilates or yoga class alone. (Also see page 203).

- **Zumba.** These Latin-dance-inspired classes have become very popular because they're high-energy and lots of fun, but they also give you a surprisingly high-intensity workout.

Exercise More Than Your Fingers

Can't make it the gym and looking for a way to work out at home? You have more options than ever before. Check your local library for exercise videos you can rent, or look for recommendations on Amazon. If you get cable TV, channels like FitTV offer workouts that you can do at home.

Easier still, check out one of these websites for workout ideas:

- **www.fullfitness.net/**
  This site includes exercises to do with free weights and weight machines, as well as Pilates moves.

- **www.fitclick.com/exercise_program**
  You'll find thousands of free exercise routines on this site; you can also connect with other users for additional workout motivation.

- **www.borkoutBox.com/workouts/**
  This site lets you customize programs to meet your specific goals; you can also track your progress.

- **www.ibodyfit.com/**
  Here you'll find free online workouts that you can view online and on your TV and smartphone.

- **Add music to the mix.** Listening to your iPod can boost your workout, as well. Choose some motivating music (you could create your own walking playlists) and your workout will fly by. (See To Tune In or Not? sidebar on page 49.)

- **Change it up.** If you're bored with your walk, try the fun workout sometimes called *fartlek,* which is Swedish for "speed play." The idea is to add variety to your workout by mixing up what you're doing instead of going at the same pace. For example, you might walk as fast as you can between telephone poles, or jog for 20 steps every time you see someone walking a dog. This type of workout adds fun to your walks—it makes the time go by much quicker!

- **Fuel your tank.** If you dread the idea of exercising, your body may be low on fuel. Have a high-energy snack an hour or so before your workout to fuel your tank. (See page 84 for 12 Quick High-Energy Snacks.)

- **Be social.** I've mentioned this before, but sharing an activity with a friend makes it more fun and makes the time fly by. Invite someone to come along with you, or sign up for a group activity where you'll meet new people.

- **Keep your eye on the ball.** Playing sports like racquetball, volleyball, or tennis is a fun way to stay fit. When you concentrate on hitting the ball, you forget about what you're doing—you simply enjoy it. Substitute playing a sport for your walk, here and there, as you please.

- **Join your kids—or just act like one.** Grab your kids and spend an hour outside with them. Play tag, pickup basketball, or go for a bike ride together. Grab the chalk and play a game of hopscotch or jump rope, or blast your favorite disco song and dance around your living room.

- **Try something new.** Just because you've been walking for four weeks doesn't mean you *have* to keep doing that. Try swimming or biking, or sign up for a new class like one listed previously.

action

Add one fun element this week—such as playing with your kids, going dancing, playing basketball, or roller or ice skating—that can take the place of one of your usual walks.

 # FEELING GOOD

the power of play

I've been talking about the physical aspects of play, but it has an emotional aspect, as well. Play can be considered any activity that you find pleasurable or enjoyable. Given that broad definition, consider how often you play. Think you're too busy to have fun? Think again—play is crucial to our mental creativity, health, and happiness. Yet adults tend to forget about the importance of having fun.

Play can be anything that you enjoy—pursuing a hobby, practicing a musical instrument, going bowling or shooting pool, or teasing your cat with a new mouse toy. The only requirement is that it's fun for *you*. Play is energizing and helps reduce stress; it may also help make us more creative.

Many of us don't take enough time to play—or we try to multitask to make the most of our "free" time. You agree to give yourself a few minutes to relax outside,

seven easy stress busters

Play is one great way to reduce stress, but there are plenty of others. Here are seven more proven ways to unwind:

1. **Stretch it out.** Sit in a chair and slowly hang forward, letting your arms dangle loose. This "rag doll stretch" helps release tension from the spine, neck, and shoulders and increases blood flow to the brain. It's particularly effective for relaxing when you're exhausted.

2. **Tune in.** One of the simplest ways to destress is listening to music. Choose any music that you enjoy or that has special significance to you, and find a comfortable spot where you can relax, close your eyes, and really focus on it. You'll be transported from the stressors of the day.

3. **Soak it away.** Run a tub full of water as hot as you can stand it, toss in a couple of chamomile tea bags, and "steep" yourself for twenty minutes. The effects of the hot water and chamomile will relax tense muscles.

4. **Play with Fluffy.** Simply owning a pet may be one of the best ways to unwind; studies have shown that stroking or touching a pet reduces blood pressure. Other studies have found that pets relieve loneliness and may help alleviate or ease depression. No time for a furry friend? Even watching fish can lower stress levels.

5. **Write in your journal.** Take a few minutes at the end of the day to record what's bothering you. Studies suggest that keeping a journal and writing about your feelings and ways to cope with difficulties can have a positive effect on your mood and help reduce stress.

6. **Get massaged.** Massage improves your circulation and relieves tension— and it feels fantastic, too! Schedule a massage at the end of an insanely busy week, or treat yourself after accomplishing something special.

7. **Work it out.** When your stress levels skyrocket, breaking a sweat is one of the best ways to fight back. The harder you work, the bigger the benefits, so as you build the intensity of your activity over the course of the coming weeks, you will likely see more and more stress relief benefits.

but then you take your laptop along to catch up on work. You're having lunch with a friend or playing some pickup basketball when you decide to answer your ringing cell phone.

Carving time out of your schedule for play can seem self-indulgent, but the results make it worthwhile. That's why some companies foster atmospheres where play is encouraged; research shows that employees who play feel happier and more relaxed and are more productive. Even a brief play break—a few minutes spent doing something fun or relaxing at work, for example—can serve as a mini-vacation that will add pleasure to your day while reducing stress.

LAUGHTER, THE BEST MEDICINE Think how good you feel after a big belly laugh. Research is proving that laughter not only makes you feel happier but is linked with overall health, as well.

The physical act of laughing changes our body chemistry in a number of significant ways. After you laugh, your blood pressure and heart rate drop, and serotonin, a brain chemical that produces a feeling of relaxation, and endorphins, or feel-good brain chemicals, are released, producing a more relaxed feeling. Published studies have proven that even a brief period of laughter boosts the immune system.

Surprisingly, even "fake" laughter can produce these kinds of benefits. One often-cited study found that adults who forced themselves to laugh for one minute reported an improved mood afterward. While we think that we react to something funny by laughing, people who make an effort to laugh more seem to find more things funny!

Your body doesn't know if you're laughing deliberately or not—simulated laughter changes your body chemistry just like real laughter. Your stress hormones go down, the world looks brighter, and you find yourself less stressed.

More people are taking time to laugh. It may sound funny, pardon the pun, to get together with other people to laugh, but adherents say it works.

So, how can you boost your own laughter quotient? Give these four techniques a try:

- Spend time with people who make you laugh—whether it's your best friend, a neighbor, or your workout buddy. People laugh the most when they're with others, usually their friends and family—and research shows that just being around someone who's laughing makes you more likely to laugh, too.

- Keep a "laughter library" of books, movies, or sitcoms that crack you up. Save up some DVR favorites so that you have something to watch when you need a good laugh.

- Call the laughter line. Laughter Yoga by phone is free and plays about 14 times a day for 15 to 20 minutes at a time (www.laughteryogausa.com/laughteron thephone.html).

- Check out a laughter club. Google "laughter club" and your city to find one of the six thousand clubs near you.

CAN YOU MAKE YOURSELF HAPPIER? While you may think of obvious factors like beauty, fame, and fortune when it comes to being happy, the fact is that true happiness has little to do with these enviable attributes. Experts say—and research proves—that even simple things can improve your day-to-day happiness.

According to happiness researchers, there are two attributes that are essential for contentment—good mental health and positive social relationships. Good mental health means more than not feeling anxious or depressed; it also involves how we see the world (i.e., in a positive rather than negative light) and an interest in working toward goals that are important to us. True self-esteem—feeling good about yourself—means accepting who you are and not holding yourself to unrealistic standards (like being a size 2 if you are a naturally curvy size 10, or never losing your cool with your kids).

Strong social relationships are the other most important aspect of happiness. Truly happy people have intimate relationships with people whom they care about—and who care about them in return. There's a health bonus, as well—research confirms that the more happy relationships you have the healthier you're likely to be.

Simply having a lot of friends or an extended family, however, may not be as important as the quality of those relationships—in other words, if you have a few really close friends, you may be just as happy as (or happier than) someone who has a lot of acquaintances. The key is how connected you feel—and how connected you want to be.

Another aspect of happiness is simply doing things you enjoy. If you have time for hobbies that are important to you, or you love your work (at least most days), you're likely to be happier than someone who hates his job and has little free time. Yet activities we choose simply for pleasure tend to get dropped to the bottom of our to-do list. If you want to feel happier, carve out time for the things you like best, whether it's watching *American Idol* (and singing along), taking a sunrise yoga class, making soup from scratch, or eating brunch with your best friends on a long, lazy Sunday.

Finally, if you've been accused of having rose-colored glasses, keep them on. Focusing on what you have, rather than on what you don't, makes you feel happier than people who are always comparing themselves to others and coming up short.

action

Your action this week is simple—incorporate a minivacation or play break into your day. You can use the Five-Minute Breathing Exercise as your minivacation or experiment with other ways to add more fun to your regular daily routine.

week 5 ACTION SUMMARY

 ### eating well

- Shop to replenish your healthy pantry.
- Eat regular meals and snacks, stopping when you are at 7 on the Hunger Continuum (see page 61).
- Drink enough to stay well hydrated, including at least five glasses of water and a maximum of one sugary drink a day.
- Use healthy fats (two to four servings per day) for cooking, dressings, and spreads.
- Record in your journal everything you eat and drink.

 ### getting fit

- Walk for 20 minutes three times at low to mid-intensity.
- Stretch and do strength training three times.
- Add a fun element to your workout at least once.
- Note your activity in your journal.

 ### feeling good

- Once a day, do the Five-Minute Breathing Exercise or take a minivacation.
- Practice mindfulness.
- Say no to tasks you don't want to and don't have to do.
- Create and maintain a specific bedtime ritual.

WEIGHT

....

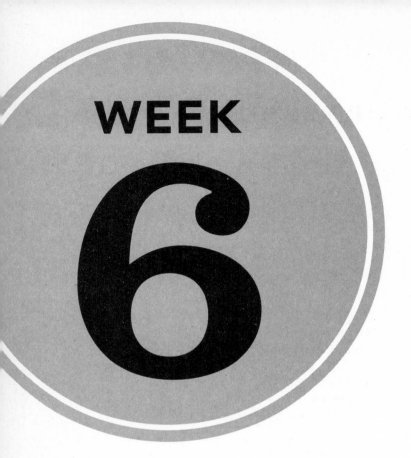

WEEK 6

this week's changes:

1. Eat plenty of colorful fruits and vegetables.
2. Walk with more intensity.
3. Try deep relaxation or meditation.

this week's recipes

The Pleasure of Produce:
Sides and Salads

- Summer Vegetable Sauté
- Sesame-Orange Spinach
- Balsamic Swiss Chard
- Kale Chips
- Mashed Potatoes with Cauliflower
- Spinach, Pear, and Walnut Salad
- Chopped Salad
- Mango Salsa
- Radiance Fruit Salad

The wealth of recipes in here is testament to the important part produce has in healthy eating. These dishes make vegetables and fruit the star of the plate, just as they should have a leading role in your diet.

summer vegetable sauté

SERVES 4 *This crowd-pleaser makes the most of summer's produce. For maximum pleasure, get your ingredients from a local farm stand or farmers' market. Serve with simple grilled fish or chicken.*

4 large ears of corn (or 2 cups frozen corn kernels, thawed)
1 tablespoon olive oil
1 large onion, diced (about 2 cups)
1 medium zucchini, cut in half lengthwise, then sliced (about 2 cups)
2 medium tomatoes, coarsely chopped (about 2 cups)
¼ cup chopped basil leaves
Salt and freshly ground black pepper to taste

1. If using fresh corn, husk it and remove the corn from the cob by holding the corn at an angle over a large bowl and cutting along the ear with a sharp knife.

2. Heat the oil in a large nonstick skillet over a medium-high flame. Add the onion and cook for 3 minutes. Add the zucchini and corn, and cook for 3 minutes more, stirring occasionally. Add the tomatoes and basil, and cook for 2 minutes more. Season with salt and pepper to taste.

Calories 189; Fat 5 g (Sat .7 g, Mono 2.9 g, Poly 1 g); Protein 5.5 g; Carb 36.5 g; Fiber 5.7 g; Chol 0 mg; Sodium 252 mg

sesame-orange spinach

SERVES 4 *Here, sweet orange segments, toasted sesame seeds, and Asian seasonings turn basic sautéed spinach into a truly special side dish. Serve it alongside roasted or grilled poultry or meat.*

 2 bunches fresh spinach (about 1½ pounds)
 1 tablespoon canola oil
 2 tablespoons low-sodium soy sauce
 1 tablespoon lemon juice
 2 oranges, peeled and separated into sections
 ½ teaspoon sesame oil
 1 tablespoon toasted sesame seeds

1. Trim the stems from the spinach, wash it thoroughly, and pat dry with paper towels or spin in a salad spinner. Chop it coarsely.

2. In a large nonstick skillet, heat the oil over a medium flame. Add the spinach in 2 or 3 batches, cooking each batch until the leaves are wilted. When all the spinach has wilted, stir in the soy sauce and lemon juice, and let simmer for about 3 minutes.

3. Chop the orange sections into bite-size pieces. Add them to the spinach and cook for 1 more minute. Stir in the sesame oil and sprinkle with sesame seeds.

Calories 130; Fat 5.6 g (Sat .5 g, Mono 2.6 g, Poly 1.7 g); Protein 6.2 g; Carb 16 g; Fiber 6 g; Chol 0 mg; Sodium 400 mg

balsamic swiss chard

SERVES 4 *Swiss chard is tender and mild in flavor, one of my favorite green leafy vegetables. You can use the basic green variety, but for extra appeal, look for yellow and red chard, too. If you like, you can substitute spinach or kale for chard.*

1 large bunch Swiss chard (about 1½ pounds)
1 tablespoon olive oil
1 garlic clove, minced
3 tablespoons low-sodium chicken broth
1 tablespoon balsamic vinegar
Salt and freshly ground black pepper to taste

1. Wash the Swiss chard thoroughly. Tear the leaves from the thick stalks, chop the stalks into small pieces, and put aside. Then cut the leaves crosswise into ½-inch-wide ribbons.

2. Heat the oil in a large pot over a medium-low flame. Add the chopped stalks and sauté for about 2 minutes, until they soften slightly. Stir in the garlic and sauté for 1 minute more. Add the leaves and stock. Cover and cook for about 4 minutes. Add the vinegar and salt and pepper to taste.

Calories 70; Fat 3.8 g (Sat .5 g, Mono 2.6 g, Poly .4 g); Protein 3.3 g; Carb 7.8 g; Fiber 2.7 g; Chol .2 mg; Sodium 370 mg

kale chips

SERVES 4 *These crunchy, addictive chips will have your whole family begging for more kale. They are wonderful served alongside sandwiches, on their own as an afternoon snack, or crumbled atop salads.*

Cooking spray
1 small bunch kale (about ½ pound)
1 tablespoon olive oil
¼ teaspoon garlic powder
¼ teaspoon salt

1. Preheat the oven to 350°F. Spray two baking trays with cooking spray. Remove the center rib and stems from each kale leaf and discard. Tear or cut the leaves into bite-size pieces, about 2 to 3 inches wide. Wash the kale and dry it very well.

2. Place the kale in a large bowl. Drizzle with the oil and sprinkle with the garlic powder and salt, and massage the oil and seasonings into the kale with your hands to distribute evenly. Place the kale in a single layer on the baking sheets, and bake until crisp and the edges are slightly browned, 12 to 15 minutes.

Calories 60; Fat 4 g (Sat .5 g, Mono 2.5 g, Poly .5 g); Protein 2 g; Carb 6 g; Fiber 2 g; Chol 0 mg; Sodium 170 mg

mashed potatoes with cauliflower

SERVES 6 *Here, cauliflower lightens traditional mashed potatoes and blends in seamlessly. A touch of butter is all you need to make them rich and sumptuous. Steaming the vegetables instead of boiling them helps preserve their vitamin C.*

1½ pounds of Yukon Gold potatoes
1 small head cauliflower (about 2 pounds), cut into 1-inch florets
⅔ cup 1% milk
2 tablespoons of unsalted butter
Salt and freshly ground pepper to taste

1. Scrub the potatoes and cut into 2-inch pieces. Arrange them in a steamer basket and steam for 10 minutes. Add the cauliflower to the basket, and cook until the potatoes and cauliflower are tender when pierced with the tip of a knife, about 15 minutes longer.

2. Heat the milk and butter in a small saucepan. Put the cooked vegetables and warm milk in a large pot or bowl, and mash with a potato masher until smooth. Season with salt and pepper.

Calories 160; Fat 4.5 g (Sat 2.5 g, Mono 1.1 g, Poly .2 g) ; Protein 6 g; Carb 27 g; Fiber 6 g; Chol 10 mg; Sodium 65 mg

spinach, pear, and walnut salad

SERVES 4 *This hearty winter salad balances earthy greens with seasonal fruit and crunchy nuts. Though quite simple, it is far from ordinary.*

2 tablespoons extra-virgin olive oil
1 tablespoon cider vinegar
1 teaspoon Dijon mustard
½ teaspoon dried tarragon
¼ teaspoon salt
⅛ teaspoon freshly ground black pepper
5 ounces baby spinach leaves (about 5 cups lightly packed)
1 firm ripe pear, cored and sliced
⅓ cup walnut pieces, toasted in a dry skillet over a medium-high flame until fragrant, about 2 minutes

1. In a large bowl, whisk together the oil, vinegar, mustard, tarragon, salt, and pepper. Add the spinach leaves and toss to coat.

2. Divide the spinach among 4 serving plates. Place a quarter of the pear slices and walnuts on top of each salad.

Calories 170; Fat 13 g (Sat 1.5 g, Mono 5.8 g, Poly 5.4 g); Protein 3 g; Carb 12 g; Fiber 3 g; Chol 0 mg; Sodium 200 mg

chopped salad

SERVES 4 *This dish shows how you can turn typical salad ingredients into something really special simply by cutting them differently and adding fresh herbs.*

1 head romaine lettuce, finely chopped
2 medium tomatoes, finely chopped (about 2 cups)
1 green, yellow, or red bell pepper, finely chopped (about 1 cup)
1 cucumber, peeled, seeded, and finely chopped (about 1½ cups)
⅓ cup finely chopped fresh basil leaves
½ cup chopped, pitted kalamata olives
2 tablespoons extra-virgin olive oil
2 tablespoons red wine vinegar
Salt and freshly ground black pepper to taste

Combine the lettuce, tomatoes, peppers, cucumber, basil, and olives in a large bowl. Drizzle on the olive oil and vinegar and toss. Season with salt and pepper to taste.

Calories 120; Fat 8.3 g (Sat 1 g, Mono 5 g, Poly .8 g); Protein 2.8 g; Carb 10.5 g; Fiber 3.5 g; Chol 0 mg; Sodium 275 mg

mango salsa

SERVES 6 *This is a colorful way to spice up simple grilled or broiled fish or chicken. Just spoon some on top of the fillet once it is cooked and then serve. It is also delicious as a party food, scooped up with baked corn chips.*

- 1 ripe mango, diced
- ½ avocado, diced
- ½ cup diced red onion
- ⅓ cup chopped cilantro
- 1 tablespoon freshly squeezed lime juice
- 1 tablespoon finely diced jalapeño pepper, or to taste
- Salt to taste

Toss together all the ingredients in a medium mixing bowl. Serve at room temperature or chilled. Store covered in the refrigerator for up to 2 days.

Calories 55; Fat 2.6 g (Sat .4 g, Mono 1.6 g, Poly .3 g); Protein .7 g; Carb 8.5 g; Fiber 1.7 g; Chol 0 mg; Sodium 5 mg

radiance fruit salad

SERVES 6 *I call this the "radiance" fruit salad because it is so rich in vitamin C and beta-carotene, two nutrients that have been shown to help keep skin smooth and healthy. Besides, you will probably have a lovely glow just from enjoying the bright flavors.*

⅓ cantaloupe, cut into ¾-inch chunks (about 2 cups)
One 16-ounce container strawberries, quartered (about 3 cups)
4 medium kiwifruit, peeled and cut into ¾-inch chunks (about 2½ cups)
3 tablespoons honey
3 tablespoons fresh lime juice
1 teaspoon lime zest
3 tablespoons fresh mint leaves, finely chopped

1. Place all the fruit into a large bowl. In a small bowl, whisk the honey, lime juice, zest, and mint.

2. Right before serving, pour the dressing over the fruit and toss gently to combine.

Calories 110; Fat .5 g (Sat 0 g, Mono 0 g, Poly 0 g); Protein 2 g; Carb 27 g; Fiber 4 g; Chol 0 mg; Sodium 10 mg

EATING WELL

the color of health: fruits and vegetables

Think about all the outrageous claims marketers make about their pills, powders, and potions. This one is supposed to help you lose weight. That one will prevent aging and reduce your risk of disease. The other one will give you more energy and provide your body with the vitamins and minerals it needs.

Yet none of these supposed benefits could be more over-the-top than the true claims that can be made for fruits and vegetables. My ad for these "wonder-foods" would look something like this:

- Avoid killer diseases like heart disease, cancer, stroke, high blood pressure, and diabetes!

- Improve your memory and keep your brain sharp!

- Keep your skin healthy and reduce wrinkles!

- Prevent birth defects!

- Lose weight without hunger!

- Slow down your body's aging process!

- Enjoy delicious, satisfying flavors!

- Get the right balance using unique color-coded packaging!

With that sales pitch, you'd think everyone would be eating their share of produce, wouldn't you? But the sad fact is that three out of four people do not come close to getting the daily minimum recommended five servings of fruit and veggies. Why? Maybe it's because carrots and apples lack a billion-dollar advertising campaign. Maybe it's because your parents forced you to eat your peas when you were little and you vowed you'd never eat them again.

I have heard all sorts of reasons why people don't eat enough produce, from "I just don't like vegetables" to "I buy fruit, but it winds up going bad in my fridge." This week, I'll enlighten you about the benefits of produce and give you some delightful and practical ways to get more of it into your life.

NUTRITIONAL POWERHOUSES Fruits and vegetables boast so many health benefits because they are loaded with nutrients—vitamin C, beta-carotene, folic acid, vitamin B6, potassium, magnesium, calcium, and fiber, to name just a few. They also contain a wealth of plant compounds called phytonutrients that act as antioxidants in your body, neutralizing substances (oxidants) that cause cell damage and are at the root of many health problems. All this nutritional power makes fruits and veggies a mighty weapon against disease, obesity, and the effects of aging.

the color connection

How can you make sure you're getting the full spectrum of protective nutrients? It's simple—since many phytonutrients impart color to food, all you need to do is fill your plate with a beautiful palette of colors every day.

- **Red.** The color red indicates the presence of lycopene and anthocyanins, which help you maintain a healthy heart, boost your memory, lower the risk of developing some types of cancer, and help keep your urinary tract healthy. Reds include strawberries, cherries, cranberries, red grapefruit, raspberries, watermelon, red apples, red peppers, pomegranates, beets, radishes, radicchio, red cabbage, rhubarb, and tomatoes.

- **Yellow/Orange.** Carotenoids produce hues of yellow and orange. These foods help keep your immune system strong, maintain sharp vision, and lower the risk of heart disease and cancer. Go for apricots, cantaloupe, grapefruit, mango, papaya, peaches, oranges, pineapples, lemons, tangerines, yellow peppers, pumpkin, butternut squash, acorn squash, yellow summer squash, carrots, and other sunny-colored produce.

- **Green.** Green fruits and vegetables contain the antioxidants lutein and indoles. Deep green vegetables are also loaded with key minerals like iron, magnesium, and calcium, plus an array of essential vitamins. Green foods help keep your vision sharp, prevent cancer, and maintain strong bones and teeth. Eat plenty of green apples, honeydew melon, green grapes, kiwifruit, limes, pears, avocado, asparagus, arugula, artichokes, broccoli, broccoli rabe, kale, collard greens, green peppers, green beans, lettuce, cucumbers, spinach, chard, zucchini, green cabbage, and so on.

- **Blue/Purple.** These foods have anthocyanins and phenolics, which may have antiaging benefits such as preventing skin wrinkling. Try blackberries, blueberries, plums, dried plums, grapes, raisins, eggplant, purple potatoes, and purple asparagus.

- **White/Brown.** Many white and brown foods have powerful antimicrobial properties and many contain a phytonutrient called allicin, which has been shown to prevent heart disease and cancer. To reap these benefits, include white foods like bananas, dates, cauliflower, garlic, onion, mushrooms, ginger, parsnips, potatoes, shallots, and turnips.

The only way to harness this power is to eat fruits and vegetables. Despite what some pitchmen might claim, you can't bottle this stuff. Well, you can bottle some of it, but research shows that removing these nutrients from the fruit or vegetable that contains them reduces their effectiveness. And since scientists are discovering new phytonutrients practically weekly, the best way to ensure you get all those wonderful phytochemicals, both discovered and undiscovered, is to eat your spinach . . . and strawberries and broccoli and oranges. . . .

THE WEIGHT-LOSS FACTOR If all the health benefits aren't enough, fruits and vegetables can also help you lose weight. I have seen it many times. Once a person commits to eating more produce, the pounds come off. There are several reasons for this.

First, there is what I call the displacement factor. Your waitress asks you if you want fries or a side salad with your sandwich. Newly focused on getting your greens, you go for the salad. At the same time, you're sparing yourself a couple hundred fatty calories (or more!) by opting out of the fries. Similarly, if you grab a banana for a snack, you are less likely to grab a cookie—and those "saved" calories add up!

Second, fruits and vegetables make you feel full yet they have very few calories, thanks to their high content of water and fiber. Research shows that when your dish includes more vegetables, you feel just as satisfied with fewer calories. Adding more vegetables to your meals can produce slow but steady—and lasting—weight loss.

Luke wanted to lose some weight. However, he claimed he didn't like vegetables. When I talked to him, I found out that he had grown up eating vegetables that his mom had boiled until they were mushy and gray—no wonder he didn't like them! But Luke loved his grill, so I suggested that he try vegetables on the grill, which adds flavor and caramelizes the natural sugars they contain.

Luke is now a vegetable convert. When he grills, he includes vegetables like asparagus, eggplant, squash, and peppers. A brush of olive oil, a sprinkle of salt, and they're read to eat. Once he realized that vegetables don't have to be bland or mushy, he was willing to add them to his regular diet. He now orders a side salad out of habit when he eats out! His diet is more nutritious than before, and he was able to drop pounds without otherwise changing the way he eats.

HOW MUCH IS ENOUGH? Depending on how many calories you need each day, you should be getting two to four servings of fruit and three to six servings of vegetables a day. That may sound like a lot, but remember that the suggested serving sizes are small—most of us can easily eat several servings at a meal. Check Appendix A, How Much Should You Eat?, on page 291 for your calorie range and to see how many servings you should aim for.

"Miracle" Fruits and Vegetables

First it was the blueberry. Then pomegranates got all the press, closely followed by the açai berry.

Every few months, it seems you hear about a hot new "miracle" fruit or vegetable touted as being able to do everything, from helping you lose weight to reducing the risk of heart disease, protecting from cancers, and boosting your immune system. But before you buy a week's worth of the produce that's in the news, keep this in mind—all fruits and vegetables contain vitamins, minerals, and antioxidants. Admittedly, some pack a more powerful nutritional punch than others, but there is no one fruit or vegetable or, for that matter, any one food that is a cure-all.

The media and food marketers like to highlight the "latest" claims, but those claims may be the result of one small study. I'm all for trying new fruits and vegetables (most of us tend to stick to the tried-and-true, which can get boring), as long as you realize that there's no such thing as a miracle food. Your best bet is to eat a variety of fruits and vegetables in a rainbow of different colors. Then you're assured of giving your body the nutrients it needs and reaping health benefits as a result.

One serving of fruit is one small whole fruit, 1 cup berries or fresh fruit salad, ½ cup canned fruit salad, ¼ cup dried fruit, or ¾ cup fruit juice. One serving of vegetables is ½ cup cooked vegetables, ½ cup chopped raw vegetables, 1 cup salad greens, or ¾ cup vegetable juice. So a 6-ounce (very small) glass of OJ at breakfast and an apple in the afternoon can cover your minimum fruit quota, and a handful of baby carrots at lunch and a cup of cooked broccoli can get you up to par on veggies for the day.

As far as upper limits go, it is nearly impossible to eat too many vegetables. So although I recommend three to six servings as the range to shoot for, enjoy as many vegetables as you care to. I have seen people go overboard on fruit, though, eating it at the expense of other healthful foods or consuming so much that they add significant calories to their diet. With this in mind, try to keep fruit servings to no more than four a day.

NO IFS, ANDS, OR BUTS As I mentioned, three out of four people don't get the recommended servings of fruits and vegetables. If you are one of that majority, now is the time to make a change. You say you simply hate vegetables? Go back to

21 ways to get fruits and vegetables into your life

1. Buy bags of prewashed greens and have a salad at the ready anytime.

2. When scrambling eggs, add some diced tomatoes, peppers, and onions for a veggie boost.

3. When dining out, make a habit of starting with a green salad.

4. Arrange sliced apples and pears on a plate and sprinkle with cinnamon for a simple yet special fruit dessert.

5. Keep blueberries and grapes in the freezer, and nibble them while they are still frozen. This is a great summer treat!

6. Make an extra-large batch of vegetable soup when you have the time. Freeze the leftovers in single-serving containers for an instant homemade veggie fix on a busy day.

7. Add fruit to a salad. Orange and grapefruit sections, apple and pear slices, grapes, raisins, and berries add juicy bursts of flavor, color, and vitamins.

8. Go beyond lettuce and tomato—add extra veggies to your sandwich. Try slices of pepper, cucumber, avocado, grated carrot, or packaged cabbage or broccoli slaw mixes. Pita bread is great for holding lots of veggies.

9. Stash some dried apricots, raisins, dried plums, dried apples, figs, or dates in your desk drawer or glove compartment. Enjoy with a handful of nuts for an energizing snack.

10. Toss a handful of fresh or frozen chopped broccoli or spinach leaves into your pasta sauce as you heat it, or stir in fresh arugula leaves right before serving.

11. Bring five pieces of fresh fruit to work each Monday and keep them in a basket on your desk. Not only will you eat more fruit, you'll also enjoy how it looks!

12. Give your tuna salad a colorful, crunchy kick: add chopped celery, onion, peppers, and carrots.

13. Try marinated vegetable kebabs when you're grilling. Just skewer mushrooms, cherry tomatoes, peppers, and onions, marinate in olive oil and vinegar with a touch of salt, and grill.

14. Grill fresh fruit—especially delicious are sliced pineapple and peach halves. Just brush with a little oil and grill until warm. Serve with a bit of frozen yogurt and some mint.

15. Try a Virgin Mary, plain tomato juice, or club soda with a splash of orange juice for a vitamin-packed, alcohol-free alternative at a party.

16. Toss some berries or sliced banana into your pancake batter.

17. Keep a bag of baby carrots at home and in the fridge at the office for a handy crunchy-munchy.

18. Spread some peanut butter or almond butter on apple halves or on a banana. It makes for a satisfying snack.

19. Top off a romantic dinner with luscious, romantic fruit like strawberries or cherries. For maximum sex appeal, feed them to each other!

20. Take 15 to 30 minutes each week to cut up fresh fruit and veggies and store them in sealed containers. Whole melons and unpeeled fruit might rot in your refrigerator, but no one can resist a ready-to-eat fruit salad. And peppers, celery, and carrots are much more enticing when they are already washed and cut.

21. Visit your local farmers' markets. You'll be amazed at the array of colorful, delicious, and very fresh produce you'll find. Go out on a limb and try something you've never had before. You can always ask the vendor how to best serve or cook your raw ingredients.

the Healthy Pantry shopping lists on pages 35–37 and circle any vegetable that you even remotely like—or that you haven't tried. Even the most ardent vegetable haters can find two or three vegetables they enjoy. Once you find them, make sure you always have them on hand.

Also, make an effort each week to try one new veggie, or a new way of cooking or preparing it. Some of your dislike may be from past prejudices or assumptions from childhood. Our tastes can change—give yourself a chance to find out. For example, you may detest cooked spinach but enjoy a spinach salad. And veggies

Eating Local

"Eating local" means different things to different people, but the idea is that you try to choose foods that are grown and/or produced near your home. (The term *locavore*, which was chosen by the *New Oxford American Dictionary* as the word of the year in 2007, refers to those who eat food harvested from a specific area, typically a 100-mile radius.) What you have easy access to will depend on where you live, but there are more ways than ever before to eat local and support the environment and your area farmers, as well.

In addition to farmers' markets, community supported agriculture (CSA) programs are a great way to eat more local food. With a CSA, you support a local farm by paying a relatively small sum of money and, in many cases, bartering a certain number of hours of farm chores for a "share" of its harvest. Then you receive the freshest food from the farm throughout the growing season distributed either at a central community location such as a church or school or at the farm itself. There are currently more than four thousand CSAs throughout the country, and more all the time; visit www.localharvest.org/ to search for local farmers' markets, farms, and CSAs near you. There is no better way to shop than directly with the people growing your food. You not only gain a better understanding of how your food is produced, you wind up with food that is picked at the peak of ripeness and doesn't have to spend lots of time in transit, so it generally has more nutrients and tastes better. Many CSAs also offer cooking classes, foraging trips, and have educational newsletters with recipes and gardening tips.

Finally, you can also find locally grown foods at your market or grocery store; look for signs that indicate the food came from a local or regional farmer or producer.

like carrots can be eaten raw, served with a low-fat dip or dressing, cooked with a little brown sugar, or used in soup.

Sneaking vegetables into foods you already like is another option. Stir a tablespoon of canned pumpkin into your oatmeal, add finely grated carrot to your pasta sauce or extra vegetables to your chicken noodle soup. Also try my Chipotle Turkey Meat Loaf on page 254, which has a whole small zucchini shredded into it. This strategy is especially handy to use with kids who resist vegetables.

If you find that fresh produce winds up getting spoiled before you get to it, no problem: frozen and canned produce are healthy choices and an easy way to keep fruits and veggies at your fingertips. Stock up on frozen spinach, peas, corn, broccoli, squash, and fruit. Vegetable medleys make for a quick and easy stir-fry, and you can whip up a frothy smoothie in no time with frozen fruits. Canned tomatoes, pumpkin, corn, peas, pineapple, and mandarin oranges are staples in my cupboard. Whenever possible, opt for low-sodium varieties and fruit in its own juice, rather than in syrup, to keep salt and sugar consumption low.

WHAT ABOUT JUICE? If you're trying to get more fruits and vegetables into your diet, you may think that juice is an easy way to accomplish your goal. That's true in a sense, but I suggest you focus more on "whole" fruits and veggies instead.

Why? Fruit juices are high in calories yet low in fiber and easy to overconsume. A small juice at a typical juice bar is 16 ounces—nearly three servings of fruit right there—sipped in seconds. If you're trying to cut calories, replacing the juice you drink with a solid version (for example, an orange for OJ or apple for apple juice) will make a difference. It will give you valuable fiber and you will consume fewer calories, because you won't be eating three oranges in one sitting.

If you're really craving a fruity drink try diluting your juice with plain or sparkling water, or unsweetened tea. But many juices also contain added sugar; check the label for "100% juice" or "no sugar added" to make sure you're getting juice alone. ("Fruit drinks" may contain little actual fruit juice, so again, read labels carefully.)

While fruit juices that contain vegetable juice (with the fruit juices masking the taste of the veggies) are growing in popularity, I'd rather see people eat actual vegetables instead. These blended juices may contain some vegetable juice but don't offer the spectrum of vitamins and nutrients that a mix of actual vegetables does. So, in a pinch, a glass of fruit or vegetable juice is better than no produce at all—but opt for the whole fruit or veggie whenever you can.

action

Eat *at least* two servings of fruit and three servings of vegetables every day.

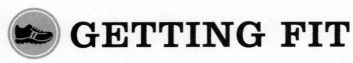

GETTING FIT

speeding up

You're beginning Week 6, which means you're nearly halfway through the program! At this point, you're walking regularly and doing strengthening and stretching exercises three times a week. This week I'm going to focus on intensity and show you how to make walking or any other cardiovascular exercise more challenging—and increase the benefits you get from it.

OTHER WALKING TECHNIQUES If you spend time outside, you've probably seen someone "race walking" or "power walking." Race walkers don't just walk—they walk *fast*. They swivel their hips and pump their arms as they walk to achieve maximum speed. (I know, it looks silly—but it's a killer workout!)

Power walking is a more generic term that can describe any kind of walking done at a more aggressive pace than an easy stroll. Power walkers take on additional obstacles like hills to make their walks tougher, or use weighed vests, hand weights, or even walking poles to increase the intensity of the workout. (By the way, please don't walk with ankle weights on—you're much more likely to suffer an injury. Light hand or wrist weights or weighted vests are a safer option if you want to increase the intensity.)

Finally, there's running or jogging. Actually, walking at a fast pace burns as many calories per minute as slow jogging, so there's no reason to run unless you want to. If you're new to exercise, though, a walking routine is safer—there's less pounding and impact on your feet and legs. (I'll show you how to start jogging in Week 10.)

WHY WALK FASTER? Back in Week 2, I introduced you to the idea of exercise intensity. Let's review the three levels:

- Level 1, low-intensity walking, is relatively slow yet purposeful. This type of exercise helps to build stamina and cardiovascular strength, and serves as an excellent fitness walk for beginners. At low intensity, you'll average about three miles per hour and cover one mile in about 20 minutes. You will feel like you are at a 5 or 6 on the Perceived Exertion Scale (page 70).

- Level 2, mid-intensity walking, is at a brisker pace; the walker typically moves at about four miles per hour and covers a mile in about 15 minutes. This will feel like a 6 or 7 on the Perceived Exertion Scale.

- Level 3, high-intensity walking, is very fast and may include periods of jogging or running. You'll be zipping along at about five miles per hour and cover a mile in about 12 minutes and feel like you are between 7 and 9 on the Perceived Exertion Scale. This form of walking is great for burning calories and toning muscles.

This week, you'll take your walking up a notch by increasing the intensity. Don't worry—you already have five weeks of regular training under your belt, so

Your Secret Fitness Weapon

Today smartphones are as common as wristwatches, and that's great news for your fitness program. High-tech phones like the iPhone, the Droid, and the BlackBerry have a slew of applications, or apps, that can help you track your caloric intake, stay motivated to work out, or add something new to your fitness routine. Here are some of the ones that I recommend (all are free or one or two dollars):

- **Fooducate.** This is one of my favorite apps; you use it to scan the barcode of a packaged food and it will tell you more about that food's nutritional value. It can help you make healthier choices.

- **iFitness.** This comprehensive app includes instructions and videos for more than three hundred exercises; you can also track your progress and store it in your profile.

- **www.livestrong.com** If you want to take a closer look at exactly how many calories you're consuming, this calorie tracker app contains more than 620,000 different foods!

- **Lose It!** Another app that lets you track your calories and log your exercise to help you lose weight—and it's free.

- **Nutrition Menu.** This calorie-counting app lets you keep track of what you're eating and how much water you've consumed, as well as letting you calculate how many calories you burn each day.

- **Water Your Body.** This app lets you track how much fluid you're consuming and may help you up your water intake.

you should be ready for this next level. In fact, you may feel that your walks have started to feel too easy or that you've increased your walking speed without even meaning to.

Do you remember from Week 2 that there are three basic ways to make exercise more challenging? You can increase the amount of time you exercise, increase the number of times each week you exercise, or increase your speed or effort level. All place additional challenges on your body, which helps you become fitter.

Why bother to do this? Because without increasing the intensity or the challenge placed on it, your body adjusts to the demands being placed on it and plateaus. Walking three times a week for 20 minutes will improve your fitness if you're sedentary, but who wants the bare minimum? Making it a little bit harder makes the payoff bigger, too. In other words, upping the intensity will increase the rewards you receive from exercise.

You have three ways to make your walk more challenging. Pick one to add a little extra challenge to your walks this week—or try each:

- Walk for 30 minutes (instead of 20).

- Walk for 20 minutes at a faster pace.

- Walk for 20 minutes at your current pace, but do it up and down hills (or use an incline setting on the treadmill) to increase your effort.

action

Your basic exercise routine stays the same—you'll continue walking three times this week and performing your strength and stretching exercises, but you'll rev up the intensity of your walks.

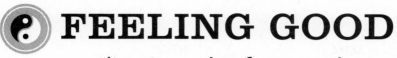

FEELING GOOD

meditation: the fast track to relaxation

Over the past five weeks, you've been paying more attention to the way you breathe with the Five-Minute Breathing Exercise. You may have noticed that you're more aware of your inhalations and exhalations, and discovered that simply slowing down, focusing on your breath, helps you relax. This week we'll take that relaxing effect a step further and explore meditation.

Meditation is difficult to describe, but it's considered an alert, focused state of mind where you are aware of what is happening around you without losing yourself in thoughts or daydreams. Usually people meditate by sitting quietly and focusing on their breath, or a word or phrase, but meditation can also be performed walking or standing. It's a way of quieting that internal and external chatter that you probably hear all day. When you meditate, you lower your blood pressure and heart rate, and reduce stress—those physical benefits are what attract many people to meditation. It also reduces the amount of cortisol and other stress hormones your body produces, which may help prevent weight gain.

About 1 in 10 Americans have tried meditation, which can improve a variety of health conditions including depression, anxiety, asthma, insomnia, pain, and high blood pressure. Even if you don't have a health condition, meditation produces a cascade of positive physiological and psychological changes that can improve your overall well-being.

Ready to give it a try? Don't be nervous—meditation is nothing more than a form of mental self-control. It occurs when your mind is so focused on what you're doing that the constant inner mental chatter fades away. There are different ways to meditate, and I've included three of the simplest below.

BREATHING MEDITATION This is one of the simplest ways to meditate. It's also a natural progression from the Five-Minute Breathing Exercise. Choose a quiet place where you won't be disturbed, and seat yourself comfortably. (Don't lie down—you may wind up falling asleep.) Breathe slowly, and count your breaths as you exhale: "inhale—one, inhale—two, inhale—three, inhale—four," and then start over at one. Focus only on your breathing, and try not to lose count.

If you do lose count, or you find yourself thinking about other things, simply return your focus to your breathing. Don't worry about how many times you lose track or are distracted by other thoughts. You can acknowledge a thought and then return your focus to your breathing. You may be surprised at how difficult you find this, especially at the beginning. Try setting a timer or stopwatch for 10 minutes, and work your way up to 20 minutes of meditation.

WORD MEDITATION Sit comfortably in a quiet place, and repeat a word or phrase over and over to keep your mind from wandering. You might use a word like "relax," "calm," "peace," or "still." If your mind strays, simply return to your word and concentrate on it. You may find it easier to connect your breath with the word (for example, saying or thinking "peace" with each inhale) to create a gentle, relaxed rhythm.

HEARTBEAT MEDITATION Sit comfortably, with your hand over your heart or fingers over your pulse. After you locate your heartbeat, sit and count each beat to 4, as you've been doing with your breaths. If you lose track, simply start over.

WOW, MEDITATION TAKES WORK! With any form of meditation, try not to let your mind wander or let other thoughts intrude. If thoughts creep in, notice them and then return your focus to your breath, heartbeat, or word. When you notice physical sensations—say, an itchy palm or pins-and-needles sensation from sitting too long—try to return your focus to your thoughts. If the physical sensation persists, change position or scratch the itch, and then return your focus; your physical body should be comfortable to slip into meditation.

Meditation is surprisingly difficult for most people. You may find it impossible to quiet your mind or that you start thinking of all the (more important) things you could be doing while you're sitting there trying to meditate! Or you may feel frustrated that it isn't working for you the way you had hoped. Try not to let emotions intrude while you're meditating—if you think of something else, simply bring your attention back to your breath, or the word you're repeating, or your heartbeat. It may help to imagine putting those emotions or thoughts into balloons and letting them float away.

Though anyone can learn to meditate, it does take practice. You're not competing with anyone else as you meditate, and you're not being graded on your performance—you're simply exploring a new way to quiet your mind and achieve greater serenity. Try it several times before you decide it's not for you—the more you do it, the easier it becomes to slip into a deeply relaxed, meditative state.

action

Experiment with meditation by doing a meditation exercise for 10 to 15 minutes at least once this week.

week 6 ACTION SUMMARY

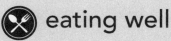 **eating well**

- Shop to replenish your healthy pantry.
- Eat regular meals and snacks, stopping when you are at 7 on the Hunger Continuum (see page 61).
- Drink enough to stay well hydrated, including at least five glasses of water and a maximum of one sugary drink a day.
- Use healthy fats for cooking, dressings, and spreads.
- Eat two to four servings of fruit and three to six servings of vegetables each day.
- Record in your journal everything you eat and drink.

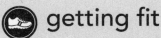 **getting fit**

- Walk for 20 to 30 minutes three times at mid-intensity.
- Stretch and do strength training three times.
- Add a fun element to your fitness program.
- Note your activity in your journal.

feeling good

- Do the Five-Minute Breathing Exercise or take a minivacation once a day.
- Practice mindfulness.
- Say no to tasks you don't want to and don't have to do.
- Keep up your bedtime ritual.
- Do a deep-relaxation or meditation exercise at least once.

WEIGHT

....

THE HALFWAY POINT

You're halfway there! Congratulations!

Look how far you've come. First, your eating has improved—at this point, you're keeping Usually foods on hand, eating intuitively, eating regularly throughout the day, and consuming the right amounts and kinds of fats, fluids, fruits, and vegetables. In the weeks to follow, you'll learn more ways to improve the way you eat and reach your nutritional goals, whether it's to lose weight, be healthier, have more energy—or all of the above!

Fitness-wise, you've established a regular workout program of walking three times a week for 20 to 30 minutes at mid-intensity, and you're performing stretching and strengthening exercises, as well. Best of all, you've learned how to make fitness fun. For the remainder of the program, you'll learn ways to further enhance your fitness level, keep yourself challenged and motivated, and integrate physical activity into your daily life.

The core mind-spirit program is established now, too. You're doing the Five-Minute Breathing Exercise and practicing mindfulness throughout the day. You've established a bedtime ritual for yourself and are managing your time by turning down things you don't want to or don't have to do—and you're including more fun, enjoyable activities in your life. You'll continue to practice these skills for the remainder of the program, but from this point on, the Feeling Good elements are optional.

Let me explain why. My intent is to make this a doable, manageable program that you can keep up no matter how crazy your life gets—not to overwhelm you with additional responsibilities. If you'd like to try all six action steps from the Feeling Good sections over the next six weeks, that's great—but if you'd prefer to implement only some of them, that's fine, too. My hope is that you'll choose at least three that you think you'll get the most benefit from. If you'd like to simplify your life, tackling a clutter-clearing project next week may be the impetus you need to get started; or if you haven't spent much quality time with your mate, Week 9's Feeling Good action step may give you the perfect excuse to plan a special date out.

So, how are you doing? How do you feel? Are you happier after the changes you've made? What additional improvements would you like to make? Take this opportunity to take a look at your Food and Exercise Journal and review your progress. Are you pleased with your accomplishments, or do you see that you've slacked off on some of the components of the program and need to recommit to it?

Let me emphasize that you don't have to have been "perfect" to have suc-ceeded so far. What's important isn't perfection but sticking with it. That means when you miss a walk or eat too much at a meal, you don't give up—you simply continue on with the program. Forget the "all or nothing" mind-set—in real life, and in this program, you simply do the best you can. And if that's not perfect, it's fine. There is no such thing as "perfect" in life anyway. What matters is that you are still moving in the right direction and facing each day as an opportunity to improve.

If you're having trouble staying motivated, try these suggestions:

- Reread your "Dear Me" letter to remind yourself of why you want to make changes in your life.

- Read through your Food and Exercise Journal to discover how far you've come.

- Make a list of the changes you've seen since you started six weeks ago. Do you have more energy? Are your clothes looser? Do you feel less anxious? Carry these with you to remind you of your progress.

- Note which areas of the plan you find most challenging and review the charts, recipes, and other support materials in the corresponding chapters. Perhaps revisiting them will spark an inspiration or solution.

- Talk to your partner or a close friend. Ask for support—can he or she check in with you regularly to see how you're progressing?

- Treat yourself to something special for making it this far—and make the treat non–food related: maybe a new shirt, a new CD, a manicure, or something you need for your favorite hobby, perhaps new scrapbooking tools or fishing gear? Hitting the halfway point deserves some celebrating!

YOUR BACKUP PLAN If you've completely fallen by the wayside, you may need more than simply a quick review of your "Dear Me" letter. Maybe you've got-ten sick and have been barely able to leave your bed, much less walk three times a week. Or you've faced a family crisis or been traveling and found it impossible to eat as healthfully as you want. Now you're short on motivation and long on guilt, and you're tempted to throw in the towel because even this 12-Week Wellness Plan seems overwhelming.

Before you give up, recognize that setbacks are inevitable. Everyone has them. What sets apart those people who succeed at changing their lives is that instead of getting derailed by setbacks, they implement a backup plan. You should do the same.

If you've been unable to exercise three times a week, for example, your Plan B might be to exercise once a week—or to simply get up more often at work and walk around the office. Can't make all the dietary changes? Focus instead on one or two—like drinking more water, eating more fruits and vegetables, or paying attention to portion size. Instead of focusing on all the things you're not doing, focus on what you can do—and don't beat yourself up because you've "failed."

One of the best ways to stay on track regardless of obstacles is to let go of blame and give yourself credit for what you are doing. Feeling guilty doesn't get you anywhere. I know it can be tough to change habits that may have been ingrained for years, and some people have an easier time changing their lifestyles than others do. But if you can continue to focus on small changes, you will still continue to improve your health. Be patient and don't jump back into the program full strength until you're ready to do so. Remember, even the smallest changes add up to big results!

WEEK

7

this week's changes

1. Start reading the ingredients list on food labels.

2. Add core exercises to your workout.

3. Tackle a clutter-clearing project (optional).

this week's recipes
Naturally Brilliant Color

- Mango-Raspberry Ice Pops
- Poached Pears in Red Wine Sauce
- Yellow Curry Dip

This week, as you begin to read labels and tune in to all the additives used in food, one thing you will find is how pervasive artificial food dyes are. Luckily, as these enticing recipes demonstrate, you can give your food gorgeous, alluring color using healthy, natural ingredients.

mango-raspberry ice pops

SERVES 4 *Like all children, my daughter is magnetically attracted to colorful foods—the brighter the better. These pops were my answer to her pleas for the artificially multicolored ices sold by vendors in the park. One taste of these brilliant beauties and she never asked for the others again. How nice that these eye-catching treats also provide plenty of vitamin C, vitamin A, and fiber.*

1 tablespoon honey, plus 3 additional tablespoons
¼ cup boiling water, plus an additional ¼ cup
2 cups cubed mango, thawed if frozen
2 cups raspberries, thawed if frozen

1. Dissolve 1 tablespoon of the honey into ¼ cup of boiling water and add to the blender along with the mango chunks. Puree until smooth. Divide the mango puree evenly among 4 four-ounce ice pop molds or small paper cups. Put in the freezer for 2 hours.

2. Clean out the blender. Dissolve the remaining 3 tablespoons honey in the remaining ¼ cup boiling water, then put into the blender with the raspberries and puree until smooth. Strain the raspberry puree through a fine mesh strainer, stirring and pressing with a spatula to press the liquid out. You should wind up with about a cup of strained puree. Discard the seeds.

3. Divide the raspberry puree among the molds or cups on top of the mango puree. Insert an ice pop stick into each and return to the freezer for at least 5 hours.

4. When ready to eat, place the mold or cup very briefly into warm water to release the pop from the mold or cup.

Calories 140; Fat 0 g; Protein 1 g; Carb 38 g; Fiber 2 g; Chol 0 mg; Sodium 0 mg

poached pears in red wine sauce

SERVES 4 TO 6 *This easy, elegant fruit dessert is simple enough for every day but is also ideal for impressing company. The wine imparts a glorious deep purple color to the succulent pears.*

1½ cups red wine
½ cup brown sugar
1 tablespoon freshly squeezed lemon juice
1 cinnamon stick
4 ripe but firm Bartlett or Bosc pears
1 teaspoon pure vanilla extract

1. In a saucepan, combine the wine with 1 cup water and the sugar, lemon juice, and cinnamon. Bring to a gentle boil, stirring to dissolve the sugar. Lower the heat and let the sauce simmer for 10 minutes.

2. In the meantime, peel and core the pears and cut them into quarters. Add the pears to the hot liquid, cover, and cook gently for 20 to 25 minutes, until the pears are tender.

3. Transfer the pears to a dish using a slotted spoon.

4. Boil the liquid, uncovered, until it is reduced to about 1 cup. Stir in the vanilla. Spoon the sauce over the pears, cover, and refrigerate until ready to serve. Serve chilled.

Calories 233; Fat .7 g (Sat 0 g, Mono .1 g, Poly .2 g); Protein .8 g; Carb 44.6 g; Fiber 4 g; Chol 0 mg; Sodium 12 mg

yellow curry dip

SERVES 4 *This lip-smacking dip is ideal for serving with blanched or raw vegetables. Turmeric and curry not only give it delicious flavor and a brilliant yellow hue, they also provide serious antioxidant power.*

⅓ cup nonfat Greek-style yogurt
2 tablespoons mayonnaise
½ teaspoon curry powder
¼ teaspoon ground cumin
⅛ teaspoon turmeric
   Salt to taste

In a small bowl, stir together the yogurt, mayonnaise, curry powder, cumin, and turmeric until well combined. Season with salt to taste.

Calories 60; Fat 6 g (Sat 0 g, Mono 3.5 g, Poly 1.8 g); Protein 2 g; Carb 1 g; Fiber 0 g; Chol 5 mg; Sodium 50 mg

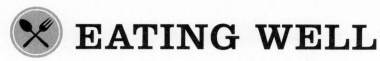

EATING WELL

subtracting additives

So many products in the supermarket boast that they're "free" of something—trans fat free, cholesterol free, wheat free, sugar free, dairy free, even guilt free—that we tend to overlook a critical question: What *is* in it? In many food products, you'd be hard-pressed to find a single ingredient remotely resembling something grown on a farm. We buy nonfat, sugar-free dessert topping because we're looking for a healthier alternative to whipped cream. But what is that fluffy white stuff anyway? Where does it come from? It may be nothing but a chemical cocktail, born in a laboratory. The bottom line may be that we're better off with the real version of whipped cream, saturated fat and all.

Companies use additives and chemically processed ingredients to make food more visually appealing, more flavorful, or more convenient. Most of these ingredients are safe. In fact, some even enhance the nutritional quality of our food. But many contribute to poor nutrition and are potentially dangerous. Two major additives, salt and sugar, are neither laboratory creations nor inherently bad, but they have become a problem because they are used excessively. Other chemical additives have been proven safe in certain amounts but are questionable when used heavily. Still others have not been thoroughly tested and are possibly dangerous. Learning about how these ingredients may affect you will help you choose your food more wisely.

In many ways, modern technology has given us safer, more nutritious, and more convenient foods. But it has also laden our food supply with empty calories and potentially harmful chemicals. The trick is to be able to make the best choices in a marketplace that introduces thousands of new foods every year. This week, we'll turn our attention to what is in our food besides the food itself, and make a habit of reading labels to make educated decisions about what we buy.

HOW OVERLY SWEET IT IS Americans have developed a huge sweet tooth. Every one of us consumes, on average, a shocking 72 pounds of sugar a year—that's a whopping 22 teaspoons or 350 calories' worth each day. Besides being a main ingredient in soda, candy, and sweet baked goods, sugar is packed into many "healthy" foods such as cereals and dairy products. Sugar not only adds empty calories, which contribute to obesity and poor nutrition, but it also causes a rise in blood sugar and triglycerides that can, over time, contribute to heart disease and diabetes in some people. In fact, the latest research shows that sugar could be even worse for your heart than saturated fat!

agave: healthy or harmful?

Depending on who you talk to, agave nectar is either pure goodness sent from the heavens or something from the labs of Dr. Evil. This is often seen with foods, where we build them up to a "superfood" status, only to knock them down (just like the media does to celebrities). But sometimes things aren't as black-and-white as they may seem.

what is agave?
Agave is made from a species of desert plants that also give us tequila. The juice of these plants is a sweet carbohydrate called inulin, which is extracted from the plant, filtered, heated, and then treated with enzymes to convert it to sugar, which is marketed as "nectar."

the benefits
Agave nectar has a relatively low glycemic index, meaning it doesn't spike your blood sugar as much as white sugar. (See Keeping Tabs on Blood Sugar, page 193.) It has a neutral flavor and dissolves easily in cold liquids like iced teas/tisanes and smoothies. It's also sweeter than white sugar, with the same amount of calories (16 per teaspoon), so you don't need to use as much. Plus, it's good for vegans who don't eat honey.

the controversy
Many agave foes are concerned because it naturally contains a high percentage of fructose. Unlike sugar, which is broken down by the body to 50% fructose and 50% glucose, agave breaks down to up to 90% fructose. That is a higher fructose content than even high-fructose corn syrup. Ironically, agave's high fructose content is the very reason it has a low glycemic index. A number of studies show that large quantities of *pure* fructose can harm your liver. However, there are no indications that small amounts are problematic.

the bottom line
While I prefer less-refined sweeteners like honey, molasses, and maple syrup, agave has its own distinct benefits, and I use it as part of my repertoire. Just remember that agave, like all sweeteners, should be used sparingly.

Let's get one thing straight from the get-go: I'm referring here to added sugar—the sugar used to sweeten food—not the naturally occurring sugars inherent in food, like those in fruit (fructose) or integral to milk products (lactose). Our bodies process naturally occurring sugar and added sugars essentially the same way—both contain the same number of calories and cause a rise in blood sugar. But when naturally occurring sugar is present in many healthy foods like fruits and dairy products, they are inherently balanced with important vitamins, minerals, and phytonutrients, as well as fiber and proteins, which slow its absorption.

I don't think added sugar is the devil in disguise. If it takes a sprinkle of brown sugar to get you to enjoy your oatmeal, go ahead and enjoy. A sprinkle here and there isn't a big deal. The problem is that so much sugar is added to food, it is hard to avoid getting too much of it. So do yourself a favor and make a concerted effort to cut back. Try keeping your added sugar intake to about 10 teaspoons (40 grams) a day—which is the amount of sugar in a single can of soda.

It's difficult to quantify the amount of added sugar in a product, because food labels don't distinguish between sugars added in processing and those naturally occurring in the food. That means the front label might claim *100% fruit juice*, but the sugar content on the nutrition label is similar to that of a can of soda. But they are certainly not the same, nutritionally.

The best way to determine how much sugar is added to a food is to look at the ingredients list. On the label, ingredients are listed in order of quantity, from most to least. So, if sugar and/or one of its many aliases—high-fructose corn syrup, fructose, invert sugar, dextrose, glucose, corn sugar, cane sugar, and corn syrup—is one of the first ingredients in your cereal, you may want to pick a different box. When you start reading labels, you'll be amazed at how many products have several sources of sugar as their primary ingredients!

SWEET ALTERNATIVES One way to go is to swap refined white sugar for less-processed alternatives wherever possible. Honey, maple syrup, and molasses are my sweeteners of choice, because they are minimally processed and contain antioxidants and trace amounts of minerals. Agave is a little more processed than those but has the benefit of causing a much smaller rise in blood sugar (see Agave: Healthy or Harmful?, opposite). Still, all of these are added sweeteners and should be counted as such toward the 10-teaspoon daily cap. Making a batch of brownies with a cup of agave instead of a cup of sugar doesn't make them healthy—they are still brownies. Enjoy them as such instead of giving them a health halo.

In case you are wondering, brown sugar is pretty much the same as white sugar, it just has a bit of molasses added for color and flavor. Raw sugar is somewhat less refined than white, but it doesn't offer any significant benefits.

DON'T FAKE IT Artificial sweeteners offer sweetness without empty calories or blood sugar effect, but I do not recommend them. Although the FDA has deemed them safe in amounts commonly used, I prefer to keep my food free of artificial ingredients. My former professor at Teachers College, Columbia University, Joan Gussow, explained it best: when asked about which bread spread she prefers she said, "As for butter versus margarine, I trust cows more than chemists."

Even the safest artificial sweeteners, aspartame (NutraSweet, Equal) and sucralose (Splenda) are not necessarily safe in excessive amounts. Saccharin (Sweet'N Low) has been linked with cancer, and many experts believe acesulfame-K (Sunett) has not been properly tested. Stevia (Truvia), the hot new calorie-free sweetener, is billed as natural because it is derived from the stevia plant, but many, including me, consider it to be an artificial ingredient because the leaf's active ingredient goes through an extensive laboratory processing to get it to its commercially available form.

Sugar alcohols, or polyols (including mannitol, malitol, and sorbitol) are naturally occurring and are added to many sugarless candies, chewing gums, and other low-calorie foods and drinks. But in large amounts they can cause gastrointestinal upset and diarrhea. Ultimately, all of these additives just exacerbate our taste for intense sweet flavor, don't offer any real benefit, and do offer possible downsides. Just as sugar pops up in unexpected places, you may be surprised at how many foods contain artificial sweeteners. They're found in everything from beverages, yogurt, ice cream, salad dressing, gum, candy, baked goods, and ready-to-eat desserts such as puddings and snack cakes. Read the ingredients list carefully—or better yet, cut out "sugar-free" versions of sweetened foods.

When it comes to sweeteners (and most other things, actually), I believe *a little* of the real thing, in as unrefined form as possible, is the best way to go—unless, of course you have a medical reason to avoid it.

A GRAIN OF SALT There is a saying that the difference between a three-star restaurant and a four-star restaurant is a box of salt. Salt certainly makes food taste better. The problem is we eat too much of it. Most of us eat 50% more than the recommended daily cap of 2,300 milligrams sodium. That's not surprising, considering a typical frozen dinner can have upward of 1,000 milligrams of sodium, and a cup of canned soup can have more than 1,000 milligrams.

The Center for Science in the Public Interest now has a smartphone app called CSPI Chemical Cuisine that tells you if a food additive is safe or not. It is very handy to have at the supermarket.

go organic, go green

In the last decade, organic foods have gained more than a toehold among consumers. Today in the United States, one in three buys organic foods rather than conventionally grown versions.

Foods that carry the "USDA Certified Organic" label are grown without synthetic pesticides, raised without growth hormones or antibiotics, and farmed using sustainable, earth-friendly methods. There are studies showing that some organic foods have slightly higher levels of nutrients, but the real benefit is that organic produce contains no pesticide residues and is better for the environment because of the way it's grown. It is also a more humane system for the animals involved in the production of meat, dairy, and eggs. Plus, many organic convenience foods are lower in additives, sugar, and sodium than their conventionally produced counterparts.

Eating organic is a simple way to not only reduce the amount of pesticides and additives you consume but to help the planet, too. Other simple ways to "eat green" include:

• Using a reusable water bottle for home and work.

• Choosing locally farmed produce, meat, fish, and dairy foods.

• Choose foods that use less packaging to produce less waste.

• Participate in neighborhood recycling programs; you may be surprised at how much "garbage" is actually recyclable!

• Start a compost heap if you have the yard space.

• Use recyclable/reusable containers instead of plastic bags for lunches and snacks.

• Use recyclable/reusable bags for grocery shopping.

The issue of whether salt (and other sources of sodium) is linked to health problems has been debated over the years. The latest research shows that high-sodium diets lead to higher blood pressure, which can lead to stroke, heart disease, and kidney disease. According to the Institute of Medicine (IOM), a renowned (and nonprofit) medical and health authority, cutting back could prevent 100,000 deaths a year in the United States, and save more people from illness.

Cutting back on salt doesn't mean you have to toss out the saltshaker or deprive yourself of flavor. Only about 30% of the salt we eat comes from salt we add to food. Seventy percent comes from processed convenience foods and from dining out (at four-star restaurants and fast-food joints alike). Prepare your own meals from fresh, unprocessed food whenever possible (as you've been doing from Week 1!) and you'll automatically reduce your salt intake significantly. Make sure to take advantage of lots of different flavorings—pepper, flavored vinegars, citrus juices, chili peppers, garlic, onions, ground spices, and fresh herbs—to lessen your reliance on salt. Also read labels to find brands of canned, frozen, and packaged foods that are lower in sodium. You may need to add some salt to those as you are cooking, but at least this way you, not the food manufacturers, are in control of it. Chances are you will add a lot less salt than they would have.

THE WORST FAT As I explained in Week 5, the worst kind of fat for your health used to be found in just about every packaged baked good on the market, in many margarines and shortenings, and in many cereals and convenience foods. It is called trans fat, and you'll recall that it has the most dramatic effect on your heart of all the fats—significantly worse even than saturated fat. Fortunately, since 2006, companies have had to list trans fats on foods labels, and many foods that used to contain them are now trans fat free, making it easier to eliminate this deadly fat from your diet. Still, it is important to be vigilant—if you see "hydrogenated or partially hydrogenated oil" on the ingredient list, skip it.

OTHER ADDITIVES And then there are the other additives—emulsifiers, thickeners, stabilizers, preservatives, chelating agents, artificial flavorings, artificial colorings . . . all with such mind-boggling names that if I printed them here, your head would spin. Most of them are safe, however. Some are essential nutrients put to good use: for example, alpha-tocopherol (vitamin E) is used as a preservative, and ascorbic acid (vitamin C) is used as a color stabilizer. Others are potentially harmful. The Center for Science in the Public Interest, a consumer watchdog group, puts out a list of additives to avoid, which I have summarized opposite. According to their reports, there is evidence that these additives are unsafe in the amounts they are commonly used, or that they are not adequately tested.

additives to avoid

Acesulfame potassium	Artificial sweetener found in baked goods, chewing gum, gelatin desserts, and soft drinks. May cause cancer.
Artificial colorings	Found in beverages, candy, and baked goods.
Blue 1, Blue 2, Green 3, Red 3, Yellow 3	May cause cancer. May cause hyperactivity in sensitive children.
Aspartame (NutraSweet)	Artificial sweetener found in diet drinks, desserts, and packets. May increase the risk of cancer.
Butylated hydroxytoluene (BHT)	Antioxidant found in cereals, potato chips, and oils. May increase risk of cancer.
Caramel coloring	Found in baked good, colas, sauces, precooked meats, chocolate-flavored products, and beers. May increase risk of cancer.
Cyclamate	Artificial sweetener found in diet foods. Linked with cancer.
Olestra	Fat substitute found in chips and crackers. Can cause diarrhea, loose stools, abdominal cramps, and flatulence. Reduces body's ability to absorb fat-soluble nutrients.
Partially hydrogenated vegetable oil (trans fat)	Fat or oil found in baked goods, crackers, fried foods, stick margarine, and other foods. Linked with heart disease.
Potassium bromate	Flour improver found in bread and rolls. May cause cancer.
Propyl gallate	Preservative used in vegetable oil, meat products, potato sticks, chicken soup base, and chewing gum. May cause cancer.
Saccharin	Artificial sweetener in diet products, soft drinks, and packets. May cause cancer.
Sodium nitrite	Preservatives and coloring agents used in cured meats and fish (bacon, ham, frankfurters, smoked fish). Linked with cancer.

action

Your action this week is to start reading food labels. Focus mainly on the ingredient list to see what the food is made of. Before buying a product, scan the ingredients for sugars, trans fats, and additives to avoid; also check the sodium content. Then decide if this is something you want to put in your body or if there is a better alternative. The good news is that by following the Usually/Sometimes/Rarely food lists, you have already given a backseat to most unhealthy foods.

GETTING FIT

strengthening your core

This week, you'll learn about your "core" and why keeping it strong and flexible is one of the best ways to maintain your overall fitness—and prevent common injuries.

YOUR CORE AND WHAT IT DOES First things first: what is your *core*, anyway? It's basically another word for your torso, and includes the muscles of your abdomen and back. While you may not be aware of it, your core is an essential part of every motion you make. It stabilizes you while you sit, stand, walk, and move, and it affects your balance and posture.

Until recently, many people didn't pay much attention to their core other than doing the typical sit-ups, crunches, or other exercises designed to flatten the stomach. For some time, however, fitness professionals have been aware of the importance of strengthening the core muscles and have developed exercises and classes to focus on this area. Disciplines like yoga and Pilates also target the core muscles.

Fitness experts say that exercising the core can help strengthen and even lengthen your spine, improve your balance and circulation, and help streamline your body. Core training should be an essential part of your regular fitness routine, and in fact it's considered "functional" exercise—meaning that it helps enhance your daily activities. A strong, flexible core is the centerpiece of a fit, healthy body.

Kate, 42, had been a runner for years when she started having back issues. After straining her back lifting her suitcase on vacation—and spending her trip in pain—she decided it was time to do something about it.

Though Kate was slim and quite fit thanks to years of running, her fitness program wasn't balanced. She hired a personal trainer, who evaluated her and told her that her abdominal and back muscles were weak. Her trainer suggested a program that would focus on strengthening her core.

Pilates

Chances are you've heard of Pilates (pi-LA-teez) by now—in fact, your local gym may offer classes in it. These exercises can help you develop a core that not only looks great but is stronger and more flexible, as well.

Joseph Pilates, a personal trainer from Germany, developed his method in the 1920s. He drew on martial arts, Eastern philosophies, and physical training methods to create a series of exercises that focus on balancing muscular strength, increasing flexibility, and providing total body awareness.

Pilates exercises all engage your core, also referred to as the powerhouse, the area between your rib cage and your pelvis that includes your abdominal and gluteus muscles. Because most Pilates exercises involve few repetitions and slow, controlled movements, you may find it a pleasant change of pace from higher-intensity workouts.

Just as there are different types and styles of yoga, there are different versions of Pilates, too. There's traditional Pilates (or Pilates, Inc.), Stott Pilates, Polestar Pilates, the Method Pilates (also known as Physical Mind Pilates), and others. All are based on Joseph Pilates's principles of flowing motion and fluidity and use the same basic moves; different versions vary in terms of their emphasis—Stott Pilates, for example, aims to restore the natural curves of the spine, while traditional Pilates focuses more on flattening the spine.

After two months of working with her trainer three times a week, Kate's back pain has disappeared. "I can't believe what a difference doing these exercises has made," she says. Kate's no longer using a trainer, but she faithfully performs her core moves several times a week. "I look at it as preventive maintenance," she says. "I'm avoiding potential problems by keeping up my new routine."

STRONGER CORE, BETTER POSTURE A strong core also helps you maintain proper posture—and vice versa. Proper posture involves a "neutral" spine, where you have a slight curve in your lower back that gives you flexibility and helps protect your back. Your stomach should be tucked in, your head up. If your core is weak, however, you may tend to slump forward at the shoulders. Check your posture several times a day—you don't have to sit and stand ramrod straight, but we tend to slump as we tire.

As people grow older, their posture also tends to worsen—weakened muscles and bone loss contribute to poor posture. But the strengthening and stretching

four for the core

By focusing on good posture all the time, you strengthen and tone your core muscles. Exercises that involve balance also target your core, because your body uses these muscles to stabilize itself. Stability balls are now popular for training your core, because you must balance on the ball while performing exercises.

Being aware of your core will improve your posture and balance, but the following exercises specifically target your core muscles to strengthen them and help prevent injuries. Proper form is important, so focus on doing the moves in a slow, controlled fashion while keeping your torso stable.

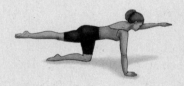

Pointer dog On all fours, lift up your left arm and your right leg at the same time, extend them out, and hold for three breaths. Switch to the other side (right arm and left leg).

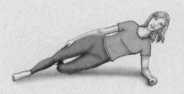

Side plank Lie on your left side, with bent legs stacked and your weight on your left forearm, elbow directly under your shoulder. Raise your hips off the floor, straighten your top leg, and hold for three breaths (or until you become tired)—your body should be a straight line between your elbow and knee. Then roll to your right side and repeat.

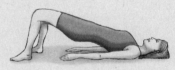

Back bridge Lie on the floor with your knees bent, feet flat on the floor, arms at your sides. Lift your hips and lower back to form a straight line from your knees to your chest, and hold for three breaths. (As you become stronger, you can extend one foot at a time to make the move more difficult.)

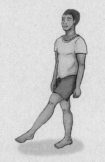

One-leg balancer Stand up, your legs shoulder width apart, head lifted, shoulders back. With your arms at your sides or outstretched for balance, lift one foot off the floor, keeping your leg straight, and hold it up while balancing on your other leg. (It may be harder than you think!) Hold for three breaths and repeat on the other side. (If you worry about falling, do this move next to a wall for support.)

moves you learned in the previous weeks and the core exercises you'll start doing this week will help give you better posture now and in the years to come. While these moves target your core, you can work this area during any type of exercise. For example, if you're walking or jogging, make sure you're maintaining good posture. During strength training, your movements should involve the core: for example, while doing push-ups, focus on keeping your abdominal muscles tight; when you do squats, maintain good posture with your head up, shoulders back, and tummy tucked in. Even simple movements like balancing on one leg for a few minutes will strengthen your core muscles.

BEAT BACK INJURIES Chances are that at some point, like Kate (see pages 172–173), you'll hurt your back—more than 80% of Americans will experience back pain at least once in their lives. Fortunately, most back pain can be alleviated with rest, stretches, exercises, and drugs to relieve pain and reduce inflammation. While minor injuries should heal quickly, preventive medicine can help forestall an injury from occurring before it happens.

Back injuries are common because of the way our bodies are designed. Our backs have supporting ligaments and muscles that enable us to stand up straight while allowing flexibility. However, this flexibility also creates the risk of injury to the muscles, ligaments, and other soft tissue that support the spine. If you don't keep these supporting muscles and ligaments strong, you're more likely to hurt your back—that's why core strength is so important. Reduce your risk of back injury by following these tips:

- **Maintain good posture.** If you sit at work, use a chair with a strong back and sit as far back in your seat as possible. Get up and take short walking breaks whenever you can.

- **Start off slowly.** Ironically, some back injuries are caused by working out. So ease into a workout routine slowly.

- **Stretch it out.** Stretching helps maintain your overall flexibility and prevent muscular stiffness that can throw your back out of balance.

- **Stay trim.** Maintaining a healthy weight will reduce your risk of injuries—carrying extra poundage, especially around your waist, increases the chance of back problems.

action
Add the core training moves to your workout three times this week.

FEELING GOOD

clearing clutter

Be honest: How does your house look? What's the state of your desk? Is it organized and comfortable? Does it take you only a moment to find anything you need—or do you spend 10 minutes every day searching for your keys? If you're overcome by clutter, there are some practical ways to help get things back under control.

One of the tenets of feng shui, an ancient Chinese philosophy of nature, is to eliminate unused objects and possessions to create clear spaces in your environment. The idea is that these clear spaces also create space in your mind and in your life for the things you want, and help reduce stress. Eliminating clutter can not only make your home seem larger, it can also make you feel calmer and more relaxed.

What is clutter? Anything you own that you no longer use, need, or love. It's everything from unread magazines to clothes that don't fit anymore to gifts you received but feel guilty about throwing out. And most of our homes are filled with it.

Getting rid of clutter is easier than you might think. First, decide it's time to streamline your life, then start out slowly. You'll find it gets easier as you go—your home is less crowded, your life feels more manageable, and you can find your keys!

Here's a simple process to help you sort the "keepers" from the clutter in your life:

1. **Ask yourself,** "Do I really need this [dress/book/CD/trinket/end table/fill in the blank]? Do I love it? Do I use it/read it/wear it/listen to it? If I didn't have it, would I miss it tomorrow? Will I ever use it again?" If the answers to these questions are no, it's clutter.

2. **Put it in a box.** You can donate these items to charity, give them to a friend, recycle them, or sell them at a garage sale. But physically remove them from the rest of your stuff—and get them out of your home as soon as possible. Otherwise, those objects tend to migrate back into your home.

3. **Go step by step.** You can't declutter your entire home in a weekend. Start off small—your desk or underwear drawer, for example—and go from there. Build momentum with smaller jobs before you tackle the garage, basement, or attic.

4. **Cut yourself some slack.** You don't have to toss your daughter's baby blanket or other object that holds special meaning to you. If your heart breaks at the thought of losing something, keep it. But if it's a sweater that you detest, lighten your load and get rid of it. Donating things you don't want and need to people who can use them is the best way to get over "gift-getting guilt"—when you receive a present you can't stand, yet you feel bad about disposing of it.

Recycle, Freecycle, and Other Ways to Cut Clutter

Reduce, reuse, recycle to embrace the "living green" philosophy, where you make conscious choices to make the most of our world's natural resources. Even if you haven't figured out your personal carbon footprint (check out www.carbonfootprint.com/calculator .aspx), buying less, doing more with what you have, and conscientiously eliminating the things you don't need will help Mother Earth.

If you've started to declutter, you're probably finding that you have a ton of stuff that you no longer want. Here are three websites that make it easier than ever before to recycle and reuse:

- **www.ebay.com.** eBay is one of the most popular ways to get rid of things you no longer want and need—and you can make a little extra money in the meantime. To get the most from eBay, include a photo of the item(s) you're offering, set a reasonable price (first check online to see what similar items are selling for), and make sure you know how much it will cost to ship the item you're selling.

- **www.craigslist.org.** Craigslist is another option, especially if you live in or near a large city. For large items, you'll have to decide whether you're willing to deliver things. (If you do have someone pick up items, make sure you have someone else with you at home. Otherwise, you may want to limit yourself to items that can be mailed.) Craigslist also has a category for "free" items.

- **www.freecycle.org.** Freecycle lets you offer household items, clothing, toys, and other usable goods to people in your community. Everything must be offered at no cost, but it's an easy way to give items you no longer need to people who want them.

If you don't want the hassle of listing your belongings online, consider donating usable items to charity. Contact a local nonprofit to ask if they can use specific items (maybe you can donate your old computer to a seniors' home or gently used toys to a women's shelter). Many charities offer pickup service and provide receipts so that you can take a deduction on your taxes. Plus you'll have the satisfaction of knowing that you're helping someone in need.

action

This week's optional action: tackle one clutter-clearing project. Choose an area of your home—and give yourself 30 minutes to do as much as you can.

week 7 ACTION SUMMARY

 ## eating well

- Shop to replenish your healthy pantry.
- Eat regular meals and snacks, stopping when you are at 7 on the Hunger Continuum (see page 61).
- Drink at least five glasses of water and a maximum of one sugary drink a day.
- Use healthy fats for cooking, dressings, and spreads.
- Eat two to four servings of fruit and three to six servings of vegetables each day.
- Check the ingredient list on your food labels.
- Record in your journal everything you eat and drink.

 ## getting fit

- Walk for 20 to 30 minutes three times at mid-intensity.
- Stretch and do strength training and core training three times.
- Include a fun element in your fitness program.
- Note your activity in your journal.

 ## feeling good

- Do the Five-Minute Breathing Exercise or take a minivacation once a day.
- Practice mindfulness.
- Say no to tasks you don't want to and don't have to do.
- Keep up your bedtime ritual.
- Do a deep-relaxation or meditation exercise at least once this week.
- Tackle a clutter-clearing project (optional).

WEIGHT

....

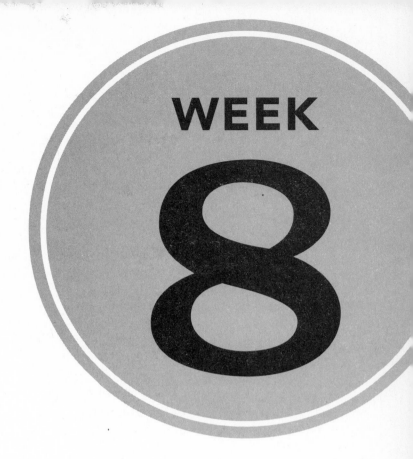

WEEK 8

this week's changes

1. Go for whole grains and limit refined grains.

2. Sign up for a fitness class.

3. Explore journaling (optional).

this week's recipes

Great Grains

- Whole Wheat Penne with Sausage and Broccoli Rabe
- Whole-Grain Rotini with Tuscan Kale
- Wild Rice Salad
- Quinoa Pilaf with Almonds and Apricots
- Grilled Corn with Lime and Cilantro
- Tabbouleh
- Baked Fries
- Peach Crisp
- Lemon Pistachio Biscotti

The recipes here are sure to inspire you to explore more whole grains. These flavorful, satisfying dishes show how you can deliciously integrate good carbs into entrées, sides, and even desserts.

whole wheat penne with sausage and broccoli rabe

SERVES 4 *The rich flavors of sausage and broccoli rabe stand up beautifully to the earthy taste of whole wheat pasta. Broccoli rabe is one of my favorite vegetables, but it has a bitter taste that isn't for everyone. Feel free to substitute regular broccoli in this recipe if you prefer.*

 1 bunch broccoli rabe (about 1 pound), washed and coarsely chopped
¼ cup pine nuts
¾ pound whole wheat penne
 2 tablespoons olive oil
¾ pound Italian-style poultry sausage
 3 garlic cloves, minced
 1 cup low-sodium chicken broth
¼ teaspoon crushed red pepper flakes
   Salt and freshly ground black pepper to taste
¼ cup grated Parmesan cheese

1. Preheat the oven to 350°F.

2. Place the broccoli rabe in a large microwaveable dish with 1 tablespoon of water. Cover tightly and microwave on high for 5 minutes. Drain and set aside.

3. Spread the pine nuts in a single layer on a baking sheet and toast in the oven for about 5 minutes, or until they are fragrant and golden brown.

4. Set a large pot of water to boil for the pasta. When boiling, add the pasta and cook according to the directions on the box. Drain. Meanwhile, heat 1 tablespoon of the oil in a large skillet over a medium flame. Add the sausage and cook for 5 or 6 minutes, until brown. Remove the sausage from the skillet and slice into ¼-inch rounds.

5. Add the remaining oil to the skillet and sauté the garlic until fragrant, about 2 minutes. Stir in the broccoli rabe and sliced sausage, and sauté for about 3 minutes. Add the chicken broth, crushed red pepper, and salt and pepper to taste. Simmer on a low heat until pasta is ready.

6. Combine the drained pasta with the sausage-broccoli rabe mixture and the pine nuts in a large bowl or pot. Serve topped with Parmesan cheese.

Calories 612; Fat 18.6 g (Sat 4.5 g, Mono 8.4 g, Poly 3.5 g); Protein 30 g; Carb 81.2 g; Fiber 5.9 g; Chol 43 mg; Sodium 885 mg

whole-grain rotini with tuscan kale

SERVES 6 *Turn a kale salad into an entrée by adding whole-grain pasta. Tossing the pasta with the kale softens the vegetable enough, while it retains a toothsome freshness.*

- 1 pound whole-grain rotini or fusilli
- ⅓ cup pine nuts
- 3 tablespoons extra-virgin olive oil
- 2 large garlic cloves, thinly sliced
- 1 bunch (¾ pound) lacinato (aka Tuscan) kale or tender regular kale, stems and center ribs discarded
- 2 tablespoons red wine vinegar
- ½ teaspoon salt, plus more to taste
- ¼ teaspoon freshly ground black pepper, plus more to taste
- ¼ cup grated Parmesan cheese

1. Bring a large pot of water to a boil. Add the pasta and cook according to the directions on the package.

2. Meanwhile, toast the nuts in a small dry skillet over a medium-high heat, stirring frequently, until golden brown and fragrant, about 3 minutes. Transfer the nuts to a small dish. Put the oil and the garlic in the same skillet and heat over a medium-low heat until the garlic is just golden, about 3 minutes. Remove from the heat.

3. Slice the kale leaves very thin and place them in a large bowl. When the pasta is done, drain it, and, while it is still hot, add to the kale along with the garlic and oil, vinegar, pine nuts, salt, pepper, and Parmesan cheese. Toss well to combine. Serve warm or at room temperature.

Calories 420; Fat 15g (Sat 2g, Mono 3.6g, Poly 4.3g); Protein 14g; Carb 63g; Fiber 10g; Chol 5mg; Sodium 270mg

wild rice salad

SERVES 8 *Wild rice is a protein-rich whole grain; three species are native to North America, and one is found in China. It has a delicious, nutty flavor and hearty, chewy texture that blends well with more tender brown rice. Enjoy this dish as a side with grilled or roasted meats or with a green salad as a vegetarian entrée.*

¾ cup wild rice
¼ cup brown rice
1 cup chopped walnuts
¾ cup dried cranberries
½ cup chopped fresh flat-leaf parsley
¼ cup chopped scallion
2 tablespoons extra-virgin olive oil
2 tablespoons balsamic vinegar
1 teaspoon Dijon mustard
1 garlic clove, minced (optional)

1. Bring 2 cups of water to a boil in a medium saucepan with a tight-fitting lid. Stir in the wild rice and brown rice, reduce the heat to low, cover, and cook for 45 minutes, or until all the water is absorbed.

2. Preheat the oven to 400°F. Spread the walnuts in a single layer on a baking tray and toast for 5 minutes.

3. Transfer the cooked rices to a large mixing bowl. Stir in the toasted nuts, cranberries, parsley, and scallion.

4. In a medium bowl, whisk together the oil, vinegar, mustard, and garlic, if using. Pour over the rice mixture. Stir to combine. Serve chilled or at room temperature.

Calories 216; Fat 13.5 g (Sat 1.4 g, Mono 3.9 g, Poly 7.5 g); Protein 5.2 g; Carb 20.6 g; Fiber 2.9 g; Chol 0 mg; Sodium 19 mg

quinoa pilaf with almonds and apricots

SERVES 4 *This flavorful pilaf is a delicious accompaniment to grilled or roasted meat and poultry. The recipe works well with any kind of whole grain, from brown rice to bulgur, but I especially like quinoa (pronounced KEEN-wah) because it has a delicate flavor, cooks up quickly, and is one of the grains richest in protein. The toasted almonds enhance the grain's nuttiness and lend a satisfying crunch.*

- ¾ cup quinoa
- 1⅓ cups water
- ⅓ cup slivered almonds
- 1 tablespoon olive oil
- 1 small onion, chopped
- ½ teaspoon ground allspice
- ¼ cup chopped dried apricots
- ⅓ cup chopped fresh flat-leaf parsley leaves
- ¼ teaspoon salt, plus more to taste
- ⅛ teaspoons freshly ground pepper, plus more to taste

1. If the quinoa is not prerinsed, place it in a fine-mesh strainer and rinse it under tap water. Put the quinoa and water in a medium saucepan, and bring to a boil. Reduce the heat to simmer, and then cover and cook until the liquid is absorbed and the grain is tender, 12 to 15 minutes.

2. Meanwhile, toast the almonds in a medium-size dry skillet over medium-high heat, stirring frequently, until golden brown and fragrant, 5 to 7 minutes. Transfer the almonds to a small dish.

3. Heat the oil in the same skillet over a medium-high heat. Add the onion and cook, stirring occasionally, until softened and beginning to brown, about 6 minutes. Stir in the allspice and cook 30 seconds more.

4. When the quinoa is done, fluff it with a fork and transfer to a large serving bowl. Stir in the toasted almonds, onion mixture, chopped apricots, and parsley. Season with salt and pepper and serve.

Calories 230; Fat 10 g (Sat 1 g, Mono 6 g, Poly 2.5 g); Protein 7 g; Carb 30 g; Fiber 4 g; Chol 0 mg; Sodium 150 mg

grilled corn with lime and cilantro

SERVES 4 *Once you have corn cooked on the grill, you will never go back to boiling it. The lightly smoky char is delightful, and even more so when doused with the cilantro-lime dressing. This is the perfect side dish whenever you are grilling out.*

2 tablespoons finely chopped fresh cilantro leaves
1 tablespoon extra-virgin olive oil
½ teaspoon finely grated lime zest
1 tablespoon fresh lime juice
¼ teaspoon salt
⅛ teaspoon freshly ground black pepper
4 ears corn, husked, silks removed

1. In a small bowl combine the cilantro, oil, lime zest, lime juice, salt, and pepper.

2. Preheat the grill to medium-high. Oil the grill's surface. Grill the corn until it is slightly softened and charred in spots, about 10 minutes, turning several times.

3. Put the corn on a plate, drizzle the cilantro-lime mixture over the corn, and roll the corn around in the mixture to coat evenly. Serve.

Calories 110; Fat 4.5 g (Sat .5 g, Mono 3 g, Poly 1 g); Protein 3 g; Carb 17 g; Fiber 2 g; Chol 0 mg; Sodium 150 mg

tabbouleh

SERVES 8 *At first glance you might think this dish calls for too much parsley, but heaps of fresh parsley define this classic Middle Eastern whole-grain salad. Bulgur wheat is quick-cooking, has a deep flavor, and is especially high in fiber.*

- 1 cup bulgur wheat
- 2 medium tomatoes, diced (about 2 cups)
- 1 cucumber, peeled, seeded, and diced (about 1½ cups)
- ½ cup diced red onion
- 2 cups finely chopped fresh flat-leaf parsley
- ⅓ cup finely chopped fresh mint leaves
- 3 tablespoons extra-virgin olive oil
- ¼ cup freshly squeezed lemon juice
- Salt and freshly ground black pepper to taste

Cook the bulgur according to the directions on the package and let it cool. In a large bowl combine the bulgur with the tomatoes, cucumber, onion, parsley, and mint. Drizzle the olive oil and lemon juice on top and toss. Season with salt and pepper to taste. Cover and place in the refrigerator for 1 hour or more. Serve chilled.

Calories 128; Fat 5.6 g (Sat .8 g, Mono 3.8 g, Poly .6 g); Protein 3.3 g; Carb 18.4 g; Fiber 4.6 g; Chol 0 mg; Sodium 15 mg

baked fries

SERVES 4 *I have to confess that french fries are one of my favorite foods. These easy-to-make "fries" satisfy my cravings without all the unhealthy fat. I have included them here because although potatoes are root vegetables, they are also starchy like a grain.*

3 large baking potatoes, such as russets
1 tablespoon canola oil
Cooking spray
Salt to taste

1. Preheat the oven to 450°F. Cut the potatoes lengthwise into 10 to 12 even-sized wedges. Place them in a large bowl and toss with the oil.

2. Spray a baking sheet with oil and place the potatoes on the tray in a single layer. Bake for 20 minutes. Use a metal spatula to scrape the wedges from the pan, and turn them over with a fork or tongs, keeping them in a single layer. Bake for 15 minutes longer, or until golden and crisp. Season with salt to taste.

Calories 171; Fat 3.6 g (Sat .3 g, Mono 2 g, Poly 1.1 g); Protein 3.8 g; Carb 32 g; Fiber 3.3 g; Chol 0 mg; Sodium 15 mg

peach crisp

SERVES 8 *Although this crisp is technically a dessert, I admit to indulging in it for breakfast now and then. Considering it is packed with fruit, whole grains, and nuts, you hardly need to feel guilty if you do, too.*

   Cooking spray
 5 cups sliced, peeled peaches (thawed, if frozen)
 ¼ cup orange juice
 ⅓ cup whole wheat flour
 ½ cup packed brown sugar
 1 cup regular oats
 ½ cup chopped pecans
 ¼ cup canola oil
 ½ teaspoon ground cinnamon

1. Preheat the oven to 375°F, and spray an 8-by-8-inch baking pan with oil. Toss the peaches and orange juice in a medium bowl, and then spoon into the prepared baking pan.

2. In a medium bowl, combine the flour, sugar, oats, pecans, oil, and cinnamon. Stir with a fork until crumbly. Sprinkle the mixture over the peaches. Bake for 35 to 40 minutes, or until the topping is crisp and the peaches are tender.

Calories 245; Fat 12.5 g (Sat 1 g, Mono 7 g, Poly 3.7 g); Protein 3.7 g; Carb 33.2 g; Fiber 4 g; Chol 0 mg; Sodium 4 mg

lemon pistachio biscotti

SERVES 24 *Swapping whole wheat pastry flour for half the regular flour in your favorite baked goods gives you both the light texture and flavor you expect and the added benefit of whole grains. My take on classic Italian biscotti is a case in point.*

1⅓ cups whole wheat pastry flour
1¼ cups all-purpose flour, plus more for the work surface
1½ teaspoons baking powder
¼ teaspoon table salt
⅔ cup granulated sugar
2 large eggs
⅓ cup olive oil
2 teaspoons lemon zest
2 tablespoons fresh lemon juice
1 teaspoon pure vanilla extract
1 cup chopped, unsalted pistachios

1. Preheat the oven to 350°F. Line a baking sheet with parchment paper. In a medium bowl whisk together the whole wheat pastry flour, all-purpose flour, baking powder, and salt. In a large bowl, whisk together the sugar, eggs, and oil until well incorporated. Stir in the lemon zest, lemon juice, and vanilla. Add the dry ingredients to the wet, in three batches, mixing just until each batch is incorporated. Stir in the pistachios. The dough will be somewhat sticky.

2. Transfer the dough to a floured work surface and shape into two logs, each about 9 inches long and 3 inches wide. Transfer to the lined baking sheet and bake for about 30 minutes, until the tops are cracked and crusty but the loaves spring back slightly when pressed. Allow to cool for 30 minutes.

3. Transfer to a cutting board, and with a serrated knife, cut carefully into ½-inch diagonal slices.

4. Arrange the slices on the baking sheet and bake for 10 minutes. Turn the cookies over and bake until golden, 5 to 10 minutes longer. Transfer to a wire rack to cool.

Calories 140; Fat 7 g (Sat .7 g, Mono 4.5 g, Poly 1 g); Protein 3 g; Carb 16 g; Fiber 1.5 g; Chol 15 mg; Sodium 60 mg

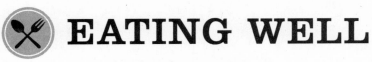

EATING WELL

go with the grain

Not too long ago, carbohydrates were the "chosen" foods. Dieters and athletes alike were eating bagels and pasta all day, often to the exclusion of most other foods. It was all part of the truly crazy fat-free craze. Now the diet pendulum has swung the other way, and it is all the rage to cut carbs completely out of your diet.

Guess what? Neither extreme works. As usual, you need to find the proper balance—and I'm going to help you do just that.

Remember that all of our calories come from three sources—carbohydrates, protein, and fat. For the record, carbohydrate is the component of food that supplies the body with its most readily available source of energy. That's because it breaks down quickly to become glucose, the body's main energy currency.

Carbohydrates are divided into two types: simple and complex. Simple carbohydrates are sugars that include refined white sugar, maple syrup, honey, corn syrup, and molasses as well as the sugars in fruits, vegetables, and dairy products. Complex carbohydrates are starches found primarily in grains like rice, wheat, and barley, and in "starchy" vegetables like potatoes and corn. While fruits and vegetables are comprised mostly of carbohydrates, when people talk about "carbs," they usually mean the starchy ones found in bread, rice, potatoes, and pasta. This week we're going to focus primarily on this group of carbs, and I'll show you how to incorporate the right amount and the right kinds of grains and other starches into your diet.

SEPARATING THE WHEAT FROM THE CHAFF If you look past the alluring claims, you'll find that many of the latest fad diets are based on cutting carbs. The promise is enticing—stop eating bread, look like a Hollywood star.

Too bad it doesn't work that way. Sure, most people would be a lot trimmer if they cut back on or eliminated *certain* carbohydrate-rich foods from their diets. But there is absolutely no reason to go the rest of your live without eating a sandwich or a dish of pasta.

For most of us, the problem isn't eating carbs per se but eating too much of the wrong kind of carbs. White breads, heavily sweetened cereals, cakes, doughnuts, cookies, and snack foods (most of which are also sugary and fatty) are easy to overeat and don't offer much in terms of nutrition. So if eating fewer carbs means you're no longer snarfing a whole basket of rolls at dinner, eating piles of mashed potatoes, and constantly munching on corn chips, great. But please, don't cut grains and starchy vegetables out of your diet completely. If you do, you'll be missing out on some of the most nutritious, satisfying foods available—foods that most of us need to eat more, not less, of.

KEEPING TABS ON BLOOD SUGAR It used to be that only people with diabetes thought about watching their blood sugar, but there is mounting evidence that keeping blood sugar in check, even if you are healthy, may prevent chronic disease and help you manage your weight. Carbohydrate-rich foods have the biggest impact on blood sugar, but some cause a much steeper spike than others. How much effect a food has on blood sugar depends on a number of factors, including how much fat, protein, and fiber the food contains; the manner in which it is prepared; and of course the amount you eat.

glycemic load of common foods

FOOD	GLYCEMIC LOAD (GL)	FOOD	GLYCEMIC LOAD (GL)
LOW		**MODERATE**	
Strawberries	1	Corn tortilla	12
Agave nectar	1	Orange juice	12
Carrots	3	Banana	13
Popcorn	4	Spaghetti	15
Milk	4	Cheerios cereal	15
Orange	5	Potato, steamed	16
Lentils	5	Sweet potato	17
Apple	6	Brown rice	18
Pineapple	7		
Whole-grain bread	7		
Chickpeas	8	**HIGH**	
Grapes	8	White rice	23
All-Bran cereal	9	Cornflakes	24
Carrot juice	10	Bagel	25
Honey	10	Potato, baked	26
White bread	10	Dried dates	42

You may have heard of the glycemic index (GI), a commonly seen measure of how different carbohydrate foods affect blood sugar. While this index can be useful, one problem is that it compares an amount of a food containing a set amount of carbohydrate (50 grams) against a standard, without regard for typical portion sizes. For example, carrots have a fairly high GI, but you would have to eat seven whole carrots to get 50 grams' worth of carbohydrate! So the GI doesn't always reflect how the food is eaten in the real world. A new measure, called the glycemic load (GL), is based on the GI but is even more useful, because it takes portion sizes into account when ranking foods—and as a result, carrots have a low GL.

When you look at the Glycemic Load of Common Foods list on page 193, you'll see that the foods with the lower GL are generally the least processed and the most nutritious—vegetables, whole fruits, whole grains, and beans. One notable exception—potatoes, which are extremely nutritious—also have a very high GL.

When choosing which carbohydrates to eat, take the GL into consideration, but don't forget the big picture. It is generally a good idea to focus on foods with a low GL, but it is also important to factor in the nutritional value of the food, and the other foods you're consuming with it. GL reflects the effect of a single item on blood sugar, but that effect is buffered in the context of a meal.

The bottom line: to keep blood sugar in line, eat whole, unprocessed grains, fruits, and vegetables; avoid foods with added sugar; keep portions small; and eat some protein and/or healthy fat along with the carbohydrate in your meal or snack.

THE WHOLE STORY Let me tell you the life story of a grain. Every grain (wheat, rice, barley, oats, and the like) is born with three parts—endosperm, bran, and germ. Intact, each grain is loaded with fiber, minerals like copper, zinc, and magnesium, essential B vitamins, vitamin E, disease-fighting phytonutrients, and even some protein. It is a proud and hearty little nugget of nourishment.

Then comes a big turning point in the grain's life. It's harvested and taken to the mill, where its bran and germ are removed and its endosperm, which is mostly starch, is ground into flour. Since most of the grain's nutritional power is found in the bran and germ, the milled (refined) flour offers little besides calories.

To make up for this loss, manufacturers "enrich" the flour with vitamins and minerals. The enrichment process helps return some potency to the grain, but even then, it is a shadow of its former self. It can never regain the wealth of health benefits it once had. Sad, isn't it? Forget "Save the whales." I say, "Save the grains!"

Whole grains with the bran, endosperm, and germ intact have some remarkable health benefits. Dozens of studies have shown that people who regularly eat whole grains have a lower risk of heart disease than those who do not. One study showed a 30% reduction in one type of heart disease in postmenopausal women who ate at least one serving of whole grain a day. More than 40 different studies examining 20 types of cancer have found that regular consumption of whole grains can reduce cancer risk by 10% to 60%, depending on the type of cancer. Whole grains also have a lower glycemic load (see Keeping Tabs on Blood Sugar, page 193) than refined grains, so they don't cause the rapid rise in blood sugar and insulin (a hormone that controls blood sugar), which can contribute to diabetes and other health problems.

GETTING MORE WHOLE GRAINS While you may not have known *all* the wonders of whole grains, chances are I'm not telling you anything entirely new. Ninety percent of Americans believe that whole-grain breads and cereals are healthier than "regular" products. Yet we're not eating them like we should. Two-thirds of us don't get even a single daily serving of whole grains, while ideally you want to have at least three servings per day.

This is easier than it sounds. Simply switching to 100% whole wheat bread and starting your day with a whole-grain cereal like Cheerios, Shredded Wheat, or oatmeal will easily put you in the recommended range of three daily servings. To take it a step further, serve brown rice at dinner, make whole wheat pasta, try whole wheat couscous, and explore more exotic grains like bulgur, quinoa, farro, spelt, amaranth, and buckwheat. Choose corn or whole wheat tortillas, and snack on baked corn chips or low-fat popcorn. Get a jar of wheat germ to sprinkle on yogurt and salad or put it in pancake and muffin batter and smoothies. Wheat germ is loaded with minerals, vitamins (it is one of the best sources of vitamin E), and fiber. Not to mention that it adds a wonderful texture and flavor to foods.

Ever the realist, I am not saying you have to eat only whole grains (but, by all means, go ahead, if you like). Personally I prefer regular pasta in some recipes, enjoy both brown rice and white rice, and sometimes I simply must have a bit of crusty French bread. What I am asking you to do is to choose whole grains whenever possible and to make them one of your Usually foods.

SAVVY SHOPPING When you are choosing whole-grain products, you have to be a savvy shopper, because many foods that look like whole grain are not. I'd like to clear up a big source of confusion right now: *wheat* bread does not necessarily mean *whole wheat* bread—it just means bread that's made of wheat. People and manufacturers often use those terms interchangeably, and it is confusing. Also, just because a bread is brown and has flecks of fiber in it doesn't mean it is *whole grain*. Sometimes manufacturers add brown coloring and bits of fiber to make bread appear more wholesome. The word *multigrain* is also misleading: it doesn't mean the grains are whole, just that there is more than one type of grain in the product.

The best way to tell if a product is whole grain is to check the ingredient list on the label. Ideally, you should find the words *100% whole wheat* or *100% whole grain*; at the minimum, whole wheat or another whole grain should be one of the first ingredients.

PASS THE POTATOES . . . AND THE CORN While corn and potatoes are vegetables, because they are starchy vegetables, I consider them as part of this grain group for nutritional purposes. What you really need to know is that they are good for you.

Potatoes are, I think, an unfairly maligned food. White potatoes are rich in vitamin C, potassium, fiber, and minerals, and they are deliciously satisfying. Yes, they can cause a rapid rise in blood sugar. But that is tempered when they are eaten—as they usually are—as part of a meal containing protein and some fat. Besides, as you can see from the Glycemic Load of Common Foods (page 193), potato's blood sugar effect depends on how they are cooked, with a more moderate effect from steaming. I believe that for most people, the nutritional benefits of potatoes far outweigh any negative, when eaten in sensible portions.

Sweet potatoes are also an excellent starch choice and one of the best sources of beta-carotene available. I always bake a few extras so that I have them on hand for a quick snack—they're delicious served cold with a scoop of cottage cheese and cinnamon sprinkled on top.

Corn is also a starchy vegetable that includes a wealth of nutrients. It is often used as a grain, and foods made of ground corn, like corn tortillas, are considered to be whole grain. Opting for corn tortillas over white-flour ones is an easy way to up your whole-grain intake.

DON'T FILL UP ON BREAD Even now, I can hear my grandmother's admonition as clear as day—"Don't fill up on bread." As usual, Grandma was right. Even if the bread is whole grain, it's not a good idea to eat the whole loaf. The main reason people gain weight from grains and starches is that they simply eat too much of them. I have two words for you, folks: portion control.

Whatever kind of grain or starchy vegetable you choose, I recommend keeping your servings to between four and nine a day, depending on your calorie range found in Appendix A, How Much Should You Eat?, on page 291. It may sound like a lot, but those servings are smaller than you might think: one serving is one slice of bread; ½ cup cooked grain, pasta, or cereal; ¾ cup cold ready-to-eat cereal; ½ pita pocket; one medium potato; or one ear of corn. Next time you go to a restaurant, notice that a bowl of pasta is likely about 2 cups—that's four servings right there!

Get Rid of Gluten?

Wondering if you should eliminate gluten from your diet? Here's the lowdown:

Gluten is a protein found in wheat, rye, and barley and in foods made from those grains. It is not inherently bad for you unless you have an intolerance to it, which, it turns out, a whopping 1 in 10 people does.

There are two distinct types of gluten intolerance: celiac disease and gluten sensitivity. Celiac disease is an inherited autoimmune condition in which eating gluten leads to severe intestinal damage and nutrient mal-absorption. It can lead to a wide range of symptoms like nausea, abdominal pain, diarrhea, extreme fatigue, joint pain, skin conditions, and delayed growth in children. The only treatment for celiac disease is to follow a strict gluten-free diet for life.

Gluten sensitivity, which has only recently been recognized as a separate condition, doesn't lead to the autoimmune reaction and intestinal damage of celiac disease, but it causes many of the same symptoms. People with gluten sensitivity have different thresholds for how much gluten they can tolerate. If you suspect you are gluten intolerant, it is critical that you go to the doctor for a diagnosis before you make any changes to your diet. If you avoid gluten prior to the test, it could lead to a faulty result.

Don't bother going on a gluten-free diet to lose weight, as many popular diet plans will have you do. Gluten-free foods are not inherently healthier or lower in calories. In fact, many gluten-free products have a lot of added starches and gums to compensate for the lack of gluten. For a healthy gluten-free breakfast see Hearty Multigrain Gluten-Free Pancakes page 81.

And a New York–style bagel is the equivalent of four slices of bread. With servings like that, it is easy to overeat if you're not careful.

action

Your mission this week is to get at least three servings of whole grains a day, and keep your total servings of grains (bread, rice, pasta, crackers, etc.) and starchy vegetables (corn and potatoes) to between four and nine servings, depending on your calorie range (see page 291).

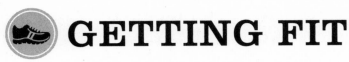

GETTING FIT

exercise your options

This week you'll learn how exercise classes can add variety and fun to your regular workout routine. Maybe you're already a fan, but even if you've never taken a class before or prefer to work out alone, group workouts can be a great way to add something new to the mix.

I'd never taken an indoor cycling class (aka "Spinning") before, and while I was curious about it I was also a bit intimidated, until I went with a friend who showed me the ropes. Now I do it regularly and love it! Here are six excellent reasons to "get with the group":

- **It reinforces your motivation.** If you're like most people, you struggle to find the time to exercise—or have a hard time making it to the gym. In a class setting, you're surrounded by like-minded people who are all there to get in shape—and have some fun doing it. That can provide an extra push the days you need it.

- **It gives you time with friends.** Signing up for a class with someone you already know is a great way to combine socializing and sweating. You may be too out of breath to talk during class, but you can head there together or catch up afterward. Even if you go solo, working out in a group is a great icebreaker. Plus, people tend to be relaxed and friendlier after a good workout. (Don't believe me? Check out the smiles on people leaving a Zumba or NIA class! See What's Right for You, opposite.)

- **It makes you more likely to stick with it.** Signing up for a class—especially when you pay for it—makes you more likely to attend. A group class also eliminates the "When should I exercise today?" question. You simply show up at the appointed time and get down to business. Left to your own devices, you may promise yourself that you'll work out "later" . . . and skip it altogether.

- **It adds variety to your mix.** Most of us are creatures of habit. This may keep you exercising regularly, but habits can quickly become ruts . . . and those ruts get boring. Taking a new class challenges your body and your mind in new ways and can reinvigorate a dull routine.

- **It reduces the risk of getting injured.** If you always do the same kind of exercise, you're more likely to develop muscle imbalances that can lead eventually to an injury. Taking different classes lets you cross-train and use different muscles in different ways, which keeps you strong, flexible, and injury free.

- **It reduces stress.** If you've had a busy day, the last thing you may want to think about is what kind of workout you're going to do. With a class, your instructor tells you what to do, and you follow his or her lead—this can be a great break if you make decisions all day long.

If you're still worried about trying something new, start by looking for classes geared toward beginners, which tend to be slower-paced and include more instruction than other classes. I took about 10 beginner yoga sessions before I signed up for a regular class; I wanted to make sure I was familiar with the basic moves before I stepped up to the next level.

WHAT'S RIGHT FOR YOU? So, which class is right for *you*? The answer will take into account your schedule, fitness level, workout goals, and personality. If your time to work out is limited, look for classes that fit into your day first, and then choose which one to try.

I suggest you think about how you spend a typical day—a workout that's the *opposite* of that may be the most enjoyable for you. If you're on the go all day, a stretching or yoga class may be a great way to relax. If you have a desk job, though, you may want to choose something more active to get your blood pumping and leave workplace stressors behind.

Visit the websites of your local gym, Y, or health club to check class schedules, and ask your friends for recommendations. If money is an issue, many community centers, colleges, and schools also offer inexpensive fitness classes for local residents. You're sure to find a class that will appeal to you. I listed some classes in week 5 on page 127, but here are other popular offerings and a brief description of what you might get out of them:

- **Aerobics.** These range from basic, low-impact moves to high-intensity classes for the fittest; patterns range from simple to complex.

- **Aquasize and water exercise classes.** A great option if you have joint problems or want a lower-intensity workout—and you don't even have to get your hair wet!

- **Ballroom dancing.** Want to master the steps of the rhumba, learn the cha-cha, or become a ballroom beauty? Look for a couples dance class; it's a great way to reconnect with your partner while you get fit. Don't have a partner? Look for classes for singles, and you'll be matched with a partner there.

- **Group boxing.** A lot of gyms offer classes ranging from boxing to kickboxing and tae bo; these high-intensity workouts are a great way to work off stress and burn calories. And don't worry—with group classes, you shadowbox, or pretend-box, instead of making contact with a punching bag or another person.

- **Adult dance lessons in ballet, hip-hop, jazz, tap, or modern.** Do you secretly dream of competing on *So You Think You Can Dance*? Did you want to take ballet as a child? Dancing is activity that can transport you like no other, and it is an excellent way to improve your cardiovascular endurance, coordination, and muscular strength. Once you learn the moves, you can crank up the tunes and practice at home in your living room, on the dance floor at a party, anywhere!

- **Pilates.** Most Pilates classes at gyms focus on no-impact mat workouts that emphasize core strength, flexibility, and proper breathing (see Strengthening Your Core, page 172). For a more involved (and usually more expensive) workout, check out a Pilates studio, where an instructor will introduce you to the various pieces of Pilates equipment like the Reformer.

- **Pole dancing.** Not for the terminally shy, but pole dancing is one of the most popular classes at many urban gyms. This challenging class is usually women-only and builds strength, flexibility, and balance—as well as confidence!

Try Out a Trainer

A group class isn't your thing? Consider working out with a personal trainer.

A personal trainer can evaluate your fitness and your current workout program, modify it to address your fitness goals, and help you stay motivated. Personal training and coaching sessions aren't just for the rich and famous—many gyms offer package discounts and "two-on-one" sessions where you sign up to train with a friend or family member. Your personal trainer will work around your schedule, but you can also ask him or her to design a workout you can perform on your own.

While personal trainers tend to focus on your overall fitness and strength, if you want to try a new sport or activity, consider taking a lesson from a professional coach or instructor. A coach can give you tips to improve your golf swing or help you with your tennis serve. Working one-on-one with a pro can give you the skills and confidence you need to continue with a new sport or step up to the next level.

Tone Up with Tai Chi

Yoga isn't the only Asian art that has grown in popularity. Tai chi, tae kwon do, kyudo kai (Japanese archery), and other arts are also popular.

Nearly anyone can do tai chi. Its slow, flowing movements are simple yet deceptively effective—studies have found that practicing tai chi reduces stress, improves balance and coordination, increases flexibility and strength, improves body awareness, burns calories, and assists in mental well-being.

Tai chi movements are performed in a position with your knees slightly bent that helps strengthen the back and improve posture. The focus is on performing the moves in a natural-feeling but slow, controlled fashion that utilizes your body weight and balance. It is both strengthening and restorative, so it makes it a good way to unwind at the end of a long day.

- **Spinning/indoor cycling.** This high-intensity workout uses stationary bikes with adjustable seats and flywheels that allow you to change the resistance while you pedal at different cadences. If you're new to the class, ask the instructor for help setting up your bike, and don't be afraid to lower your bike's resistance if you need to.

- **Step.** Step classes have been around for more than 25 years, and they're still a popular mainstay at many gyms. You get a low-impact, high-intensity workout, and most include core and upper body moves, as well.

- **Tai chi.** This gentle form of exercise and self-defense consists of slow, smooth movements and is appropriate for almost any fitness level. (See Box above for more on tai chi's benefits.)

- **Yoga.** Yoga classes focus on flexibility, strength, and balance, but not all are low-intensity. Classes for Bikram, Baptiste, and power yoga are usually quite challenging; make sure you know what you're getting into before you sign up. Yogalates (also called PiYo), a blend of yoga and Pilates moves, has also become popular. (See Yoga: The Allover Workout on page 202 for more on yoga types and benefits.)

action

Sign up for an exercise class of your choosing and do it in place of one of your usual walks.

yoga: the allover workout

More than 20 million Americans have added yoga to their workout regimens, and that number is likely to grow, especially among baby boomers who want to maintain their strength and flexibility as they age.

The word *yoga* means "to join" (as in *yoke*) and refers to linking the mind and body. Yoga uses mental focus, breathing, and physical movements to achieve this connection.

New research has proven that regular yoga practice reduces some risk factors for heart disease and may help reduce the risk of developing diabetes. It's also proven to build strength and flexibility, reduce stress, and may assist in weight loss.

Yoga instills a sense of calm and relaxation, and it boosts stamina, as well. The focus on breathing, physical alignment, and philosophical perspective has both a restorative and energizing effect. And as someone who has practiced yoga for years, I can tell you it's one of the most effective stress-management tools I know of. The peace of mind and perspective you cultivate in yoga class extends throughout your day and week.

If you've tried yoga before and weren't crazy about it, don't write it off. Classes and instructors vary widely in their approach and the forms, or poses, they use, so it's worth giving it another try. If you're new to yoga, ask about the class offered before you sign up; some types of yoga are gentle and restorative, while others qualify as high-intensity workouts. The most popular forms of yoga include:

- **Ashtanga.** A set series of challenging, energizing postures. It is relatively fast-paced and requires and cultivates a lot of stamina.

- **Anusara.** A modern form of hatha yoga that focuses on alignment both in the physical poses and with the spiritual/philosphical aspect of the practice.

- **Bikram or Vikram.** Includes very demanding physical poses and is practiced in a heated room (usually about 105°F) to allow muscles, ligaments, and joints to stretch further.

- **Hatha.** While many forms of yoga fall under the basic category of "hatha," generally this means yoga that uses the practice of asanas, or postures, to help balance, purify, and strengthen the body and that incorporates breath flow. Hatha classes are often aimed at beginners or people new to yoga, but many gyms offer advanced hatha classes, as well.

- **Iyengar.** This type of yoga puts more emphasis on form and less on breath control. It's very structured and puts a lot of attention on alignment.

- **Kripalu.** A flowing form of yoga that includes meditation. After you master certain poses, you incorporate meditation into your practice; then you practice them as a moving meditation, performing them in a continuous flow.

- **Vinyasa.** Also called flow yoga, this is a faster-paced practice where you move from one pose to the next on each inhale and exhale.

- **Yogalates.** Not a true yoga class, this style includes elements of both yoga and Pilates.

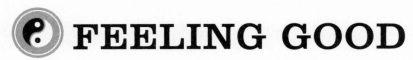

FEELING GOOD

the power of the pen

You've been keeping a Food and Exercise Journal for seven weeks now, writing down what and when you eat, and keeping track of your workouts. Simply making that commitment is bound to help you meet your nutritional and fitness goals.

Taking your journaling a step further and writing about your life, your feelings, your dreams, and your challenges offers additional benefits. This more in-depth journaling can make a difference in the way you feel, help reduce anxiety and overcome grief, give you answers to problems, and provide you with insights into your life you may not have had before.

Researchers are now finding there are health benefits to journaling. Keeping a journal has been shown to improve overall physical health, as well as psychological well-being. It may be that writing down ways to deal with problems or expressing your feelings on the page reduces the amount of stress you feel. On a practical level, journaling can help you set goals and take time to reflect upon your life.

Tiffany was a mom of 6-month-old twins who was trying to decide whether to return to work or stay home with her children. She used her journal to hash out the pros and cons of each option. "I talked about it with my husband, but what helped me was writing down all of the possibilities. When I looked at what I would be getting in terms of income, I realized that I wouldn't make that much after I deducted the cost of child care," says Tiffany, 34.

"But it wasn't just the financial aspect of it. When I wrote about it, I realized that I really *wanted* to stay home. I'd told myself I'd go back to work for so long that I hadn't realized that." After talking about it with her husband, they agreed that she'd stay home until the twins were in school.

Tiffany still keeps a journal. "I write down the babies' milestones, but I also write about myself and what I'm feeling," she says. "Sometimes it's easy to forget that I'm not just their mommy—I'm still myself, too. Writing helps me stay connected to that person."

GETTING STARTED You don't need a fancy ink pen or an elegant diary to keep your journal—a simple notebook is all that's necessary. In fact, you can create a section in your Food and Exercise Journal to write more elaborately about your thoughts and feelings if you find it easier to have everything in one place. If you prefer something more upscale, bookstores offer dozens of different journals in all sizes, shapes, and covers. Some have lined paper; some have blank paper or even graph paper. Remember, the most important thing is what you do with the journal.

Make a note of the date and begin writing. You may want to start with what's happening in your life right now, or simply record the events of the day. There are so many ways you can use this journal. There's no "right" or "wrong" when it comes to journaling.

- Get in touch with your emotions and feelings.

- Track the events of day-to-day life.

- Express thankfulness for all the good things in your life (some people keep special "gratitude journals," where they list what they're thankful for).

- Determine your priorities and goals, and track your progress toward them.

- Record your children's progress as they learn and grow.

- Write down your frustrations, and think of ways to cope during stressful times.

WHAT DO I WRITE ABOUT? Want to write but you're stuck? Give these writing prompts a try:

- Write down five words that describe how you're feeling. Worried? Tired? Distracted? Comfortable? Content? Take one of those words and explore it. What are you worried about, for example? Why do you feel content?

- List five things you're grateful for. They can be big or small—hearing your child's laugh in the morning, wearing thick fluffy socks, or feeling healthy and strong.

- Describe your setting. Where are you? What does this place feel like? What do you like about it? What don't you like?

- Make a list of your goals and what you'd like to accomplish in your life. Would you like to learn how to scuba dive? Take a ride in a hot-air balloon? Meet the president? Write a book? Swim with dolphins? Drive in a NASCAR race? Use your journal to dream. You may be surprised at what comes out.

- Write down the achievements you're most proud of. What makes the list and why? How has this impacted your life?

- Think about the people in your life. Write about how they've made a difference in yours. What effect are you having on their lives? Is it what you intend?

- Make a list of your favorites—favorite food, favorite movie, favorite book. What do they have in common? How often do you indulge in your favorites?

- Start with "I remember . . ." and write a memory. It can be anything—an event from your childhood or something that happened last week.

You might decide to write every night or just once a week, but I suggest you commit to a journaling schedule to get into the rhythm of this new habit and reap its profound benefits. Keeping your journal in a conspicuous place—on your nightstand, for example—will remind you to write in it, but on the other hand you may want to stash it in a secret place, so no one else can read it. You can keep it in a locked box, hide it, or ask the people around you not to read it. Even then, you may feel more comfortable using code words or secret names for some events or people in your life. You shouldn't have to worry about hurting someone's feelings in your journal—it should be a place that is just for you.

action

You've been keeping a Food and Exercise Journal to record your food intake and exercise program. In addition, as an option, write about anything you're feeling for five minutes a day. If you like, you can designate a separate notebook or diary as a journal and begin keeping it regularly.

Take Your Journal Online

There's another option to consider when it comes to your journal, especially if you spend a lot of time on your computer. For many people, online journals, aka blogs (originally "web logs"), are easier and more fun, offering a way to connect with other people and also record your thoughts, feelings, and experiences. Your blog can be as personal and confessional as you like; if you're uncomfortable with having others read it, you can set it up to be viewed only by you. Or you can go "public" (you can always use a pseudonym, or "handle," and open up your blog up to the world or to a limited number of select people). There are more than 400 million English-language blogs alone.

You can set up a blog in less than 20 minutes; check out www.blogger.com, www.opendiary.com, or www.livejournal.com to set up your own.

eating well

- Shop to replenish your healthy pantry.
- Eat regular meals and snacks, stopping when you are at 7 on the Hunger Continuum (see page 61).
- Drink enough to stay well hydrated, including at least five glasses of water and a maximum of one sugary drink a day.
- Use healthy fats for cooking, dressings, and spreads.
- Eat two to four servings of fruit and three to six servings of vegetables each day.
- Check the ingredient list on your food labels.
- Get at least three servings of whole grains a day and limit refined grains.
- Record in your journal everything you eat and drink.

 getting fit

- Walk for 20 to 30 minutes three times at mid-intensity.
- Stretch and do strength training three times.
- Include a fun element in your fitness program.
- Sign up for a class.
- Note your activity in your journal.

feeling good

- Do the Five-Minute Breathing Exercise or minivacation once a day.
- Practice mindfulness.
- Say no to tasks you don't want to and don't have to do.
- Keep up your bedtime ritual.
- Do a deep-relaxation or meditation exercise once.
- Optional:
  Tackle a clutter-clearing project.
  Explore journaling.

WEIGHT
....

WEEK 9

this week's changes

1. Eat fish at least twice.

2. Try some more challenging strength-training moves.

3. Plan some special time with your partner or family (optional).

this week's recipes

Easy Seafood Dinners

- Citrus-Ginger Flounder with Snow Peas
- Poached Salmon with Mustard-Dill Sauce
- Cod with Almond-Shallot Topping
- Tilapia with Greek-Style Herb Sauce
- Scallop and Asparagus Sauté with Lemon and Thyme

The recipes here highlight how quick, easy, and flavorful a seafood meal can be. If you aren't already a fish lover, try these recipes and I know you will be hooked.

citrus-ginger flounder with snow peas

SERVES 4 *Drizzling the fish with the dressing and wrapping it in foil essentially allows it to steam in the oven. This gentle, flavor-infused cooking method brings out the best in the delicate flounder. Plus, you get to steam your vegetable along with it. I like to serve this over a bed of rice to absorb the juices.*

- **4 small flounder fillets, 4 to 6 ounces each**
- **4 cups snow peas (about ¾ pound)**
- **½ cup Citrus-Ginger Dressing (page 116)**
- **Lemon wedges**

1. Preheat the oven to 425°F. Place each fillet on a large square of foil and turn up the edges of the foil. Top each fillet with 1 cup of snow peas and 2 tablespoons of dressing. Fold the foil around the fish to form a pouch and crimp it so that it is sealed.

2. Put the foil pouches on a baking sheet and bake for 15 to 20 minutes, until fish flakes easily with a fork. Put the contents of each pouch on a plate and garnish with lemon.

Calories 214; Fat 6.4 g (Sat .7 g, Mono 3 g, Poly 1.9 g); Protein 28.6 g; Carb 9.5 g; Fiber 1.7 g; Chol 68 mg; Sodium 118 mg

poached salmon with mustard-dill sauce

SERVES 4 *This dish holds a special place in my heart, as it was the first one I ever made for Thom, before we were married. Needless to say, it won him over. The creamy, tangy, herb-flecked sauce is the ideal accompaniment for the rich salmon.*

4 salmon fillets, 4 to 6 ounces each
Mustard-Dill Sauce (page 117)

1. Pour 3 cups of water into a deep, nonstick skillet and bring to a boil. Add the salmon and more water if necessary to cover the fish completely. Cover the skillet and cook over medium-low heat for about 10 minutes per inch of thickness of the fish. Transfer the salmon to a plate using two spatulas. Cover and chill in the refrigerator for 2 hours or more.

2. Spoon the sauce over the chilled salmon and serve.

Calories 280; Fat 15.4 g (Sat 3.1 g, Mono 5.5 g, Poly 5.6 g); Protein 30 g; Carb 2.6 g; Fiber 0 g; Chol 84.2 mg; Sodium 165 mg

cod with almond-shallot topping

SERVES 4 *Cod's firm, flaky texture and buttery flavor are perfect for this crunchy, herbal topping loaded with aromatic sautéed shallots.*

2 tablespoons olive oil
4 cod fillets, 4 to 6 ounces each
1 cup chopped shallots
½ cup almonds, chopped
⅓ cup finely chopped fresh flat-leaf parsley
2 tablespoons fresh lemon juice
Salt and freshly ground black pepper to taste

1. Heat 1 tablespoon of the oil in a large nonstick skillet on a medium flame. Place the fish in the pan and cook for about 8 minutes, or until the fish is cooked through, turning once. Transfer the fish to a plate and cover to keep warm.

2. Add the other tablespoon of oil and the shallots to the skillet, and cook over moderate heat, stirring occasionally, for 3 to 4 minutes. Add the almonds and, stirring frequently, cook for 3 minutes more. Add the parsley, lemon juice, and salt and pepper to taste. Cook for 1 minute more. Spoon the topping over the fish and serve.

Calories 300; Fat 15.9 g (Sat 1.7 g, Mono 10.3 g, Poly 2.9 g); Protein 29.7 g; Carb 10.6 g; Fiber 1.9 g; Chol 61 mg; Sodium 81 mg

tilapia with greek-style herb sauce

SERVES 4 *A perfect example of how much of a breeze it can be to whip up flavorful, healthfully prepared fish. It is on the table impressing everyone in less than 10 minutes.*

3 tablespoons extra-virgin olive oil
1 teaspoon finely grated lemon zest
1½ tablespoons fresh lemon juice
½ teaspoon dried oregano
⅛ teaspoon salt, plus an additional ⅛ teaspoon
⅛ teaspoon freshly ground black pepper, plus an additional ⅛ teaspoon
2 tablespoons chopped fresh flat-leaf parsley leaves
Cooking spray
4 (5-ounce) tilapia filets

1. Preheat the broiler. In a small bowl, whisk together 2 tablespoons of the oil, the lemon zest, lemon juice, oregano, ⅛ teaspoon of salt, and ⅛ teaspoon of pepper. Stir in the parsley.

2. Spray a baking sheet or broiling pan with cooking spray. Place the fillets on it, and then brush each fillet on both sides with the remaining tablespoon of oil. Season each fillet with ⅛ teaspoon each of salt and pepper. Broil on high, 4 inches from the flame, until the fish is no longer translucent and flakes easily with a fork, about 5 minutes.

3. Place the fish on a serving plate and spoon the sauce over it.

Calories 230; Fat 13 g (Sat 2.5 g, Mono 8.2 g, Poly 1.7 g); Protein 29 g; Carb 1 g; Fiber 0 g; Chol 70 mg; Sodium 220 mg

scallop and asparagus sauté with lemon and thyme

SERVES 4 *With this recipe in your arsenal, you are one pan and 10 minutes away from a flavorful, elegant meal anytime. The scallops release a lot of liquid when cooked, so by simmering them covered with the shallots and thyme you wind up with a delicate, fragrant broth to spoon over rice or dip your bread into.*

2 tablespoons olive oil
¼ cup diced shallots
1 tablespoon chopped fresh thyme leaves
2 teaspoons finely grated lemon zest
1 bunch of asparagus (about 1 pound), trimmed and cut on the bias into 1-inch pieces
1¼ pounds bay scallops, rinsed and patted dry
2 tablespoons fresh lemon juice
¼ teaspoon salt
¼ teaspoon freshly ground black pepper

1. Heat the oil in a large skillet over medium-high heat (you'll need a lid, too, to cover it later). Add the shallots and cook until they soften, about 2 minutes. Add the thyme, lemon zest, and asparagus, and cook, stirring, until the asparagus softens slightly, about 1 minute.

2. Stir in the scallops, cover, reduce the heat to medium, and cook, stirring occasionally, until the scallops are opaque and the asparagus is crisp-tender, 4 to 5 minutes. Drizzle with lemon juice and season with salt and pepper. Serve with the accumulated juices.

Calories 220; Fat 8 g (Sat 1 g, Mono 5 g, Poly 1.2 g); Protein 27 g; Carb 10 g; Fiber 3 g; Chol 45 mg; Sodium 380 mg

EATING WELL

go fish

Fish is one of those foods people seem to either love or fear. If you already love fish, this week you will be happy to learn about its benefits and some new, healthy ways to prepare it. I'll also tell you which seafood is safest and which you are better off avoiding. If you fear fish because you think it will taste "fishy" or because you haven't a clue how to buy it or cook it, this is the week to jump in and explore some seafood.

SEAFOOD: THE GOOD NEWS The benefits of eating seafood are overwhelming. A recent study published by the American Heart Association shows that just two seafood meals a week can reduce your risk of dying of a heart attack by a whopping 30%. Fish helps the heart by protecting against arrhythmias, lowering triglycerides and blood pressure, and keeping blood vessels healthy. Studies also show that eating seafood may ward against cancer, help keep skin healthy and more youthful-looking, keep your brain healthy, and ease arthritis pain.

Beyond that, seafood provides lots of nutrition and fills you up without a lot of calories, making it an ideal food if you're trying to stay trim (and who isn't, really?). It is an excellent source of high-quality protein, and it's rich in B vitamins and minerals like zinc, magnesium, and iron. Shellfish and fish like sole, cod, and catfish are extra-lean and very low in calories. Fish such as salmon, sardines, and herring are higher in fat, but their fat content actually makes them an even bigger boon to your health.

The fat in fish—omega-3—is what gives its incredible healing properties. We can get omega-3 from some plant foods like flax, walnuts, and leafy green vegetables, but that is a different form (called ALA), not nearly as powerful as the form found in fish (EPA and DHA).

SOME CONCERNS As our waters have become polluted with industrial waste like mercury and polychlorinated biphenyls (PCBs), so have many of our fish. We eat the fish, and those toxins can accumulate in our bodies over time. In large amounts, some of these can ultimately damage our neurological systems.

For most folks the benefits of eating fish far outweigh any potential downsides, and more is generally better. But since rapidly growing cells are especially vulnerable to toxins, the risk-benefit balance shifts for pregnant women, women who may become pregnant, and young children. That is why people in these categories should eat no more than 12 ounces of fish each week and should be extra careful to stick with those likely to be lowest in contaminants (see page 216). It is worth noting that seafood has many important health benefits for pregnant women and children, as well, so they should not take this advisory as a message to stay away from fish in general, but rather be sure to eat the right kinds regularly.

AVOIDING CONTAMINANTS You can avoid mercury and other toxins by not choosing the big fish at the top of the food chain. The fish highest in mercury are what I call the Big Four: king mackerel, shark, swordfish, and tilefish. These fish live longer and eat other fish, so over time they accumulate and concentrate contaminants in their tissues. Other big fish, such as grouper and large tuna (tuna steaks and chunk white canned tuna), have slightly less mercury and are fine to eat occasionally, but for the purest choice, stick with smaller fish like skipjack tuna, light canned tuna, sardines, and flounder that aren't swimming around long enough to accumulate much mercury at all.

FARMED VERSUS WILD-CAUGHT There's one more issue about fish you may be wondering about—whether there's a difference between those that are farmed and those that are wild, or fished. Salmon in particular has garnered a lot of attention because of the growing number of salmon farms. Farmed salmon tends to have higher levels of omega 3 fats but also contains more pollutants like PCBs and toxic man-made chemicals. Eating farmed salmon is basically fine because, again, the benefits outweigh any downsides for most folks. But when you can, opt for wild. And when you cook salmon, trim as much fat and skin as you can to reduce your exposure to toxins.

If you like to fish or have a fisherman in the family, you know freshly caught fish is so flavorful. But before you indulge, be sure to contact your state health department about the safety of the fish in your area.

SHELLFISH AND CHOLESTEROL Happily, most shellfish is low in mercury, but many people shun shellfish because they have heard it is high in cholesterol. It's true that some shellfish, especially squid and shrimp, is high in cholesterol. Three ounces of shrimp has 170 milligrams of cholesterol, a little more than half the 300-milligrams-per-day limit recommended by the American Heart Association; squid and crab are also relatively high in cholesterol. But the latest research shows that the cholesterol you eat isn't the main dietary factor influencing your blood cholesterol. Saturated fat is. Since shellfish has virtually no saturated fat (unless you dip it in butter!), it can easily be a part of heart-healthy eating. So feel free to enjoy it!

TO MARKET, TO MARKET You belly up to the fish counter and stand there perplexed. You are thinking, Is this a good place to buy my fish? How do I know if it

usually/sometimes/rarely seafood list

usually

Choose most frequently. These seafoods contain the lowest level of mercury:

	MERCURY	OMEGA-3
Anchovies	low	highest
Bass	low	low–moderate
Catfish	low	moderate
Clams	low	low
Cod	low–moderate	low
Crab	low	low
Flounder/Sole	low	moderate
Halibut	low–moderate	moderate
Herring	low	highest
Lobster (spiny)	low	low
Mackerel (Atlantic)	low	high
Oysters	low	moderate
Salmon	low	highest
Sardines	low	highest
Scallops	low	low
Shrimp	low	low
Squid	low	low
Tilapia	low	low
Trout (freshwater)	low	high
Whitefish	low	high
Mahi mahi	low	moderate
Perch (freshwater)	low	low
Sablefish	low	highest
Snapper	low	low
Tuna (canned light)	low	high

sometimes

These seafoods contain moderate levels of mercury:

	MERCURY	OMEGA-3
Bluefish	moderate	moderate
Lobster (North American)	moderate	low
Grouper	moderate–high	moderate
Orange roughy	moderate–high	moderate
Tuna (fresh, canned albacore)	moderate	moderate–high

rarely

These seafoods contain high mercury levels. Avoid entirely if you are pregnant, nursing, or plan to get pregnant:

	MERCURY	OMEGA-3
King mackerel	highest	highest
Shark	highest	high
Swordfish	highest	high
Tilefish	highest	moderate

is fresh? Should I buy it frozen? How do I cook it once I get home? Will my kids like it? Maybe I should just get some meat to make hamburger. Before you give up, let me help.

First of all, step back and evaluate the vendor. The area should look and smell clean. Fish should be displayed on a thick bed of fresh, not melting, ice, and the seafood should be arranged with the bellies down so that the melting ice drains away from the fish, reducing the chance of spoilage. The person behind the counter should be knowledgeable about different types of seafood and freely tell you how old the food is and explain why it is fresh.

The fish itself should have firm and shiny flesh that springs back when pressed. Whole fish should have bright red gills, clear eyes (some fish, like walleye, have naturally cloudy eyes, however), and be slime free. The fish should smell like the sea, not fishy or ammonia-like.

Frozen fish is also a good option and offers an easy way to have seafood at your fingertips. I actually prefer to buy shrimp frozen, because they are usually shipped frozen and defrosted prior to sale at a fish counter anyway. They don't take long to defrost, so it is easy to boil or sauté some up on the spur of the moment, or toss a few into a jarred pasta sauce after you heat it (I like to add some spinach, too) for an effortless pasta dinner. Frozen fillets are also a good choice. They taste very fresh, as they are usually flash-frozen soon after being caught. Just be sure to buy plain fillets, not the breaded, fried kind.

Canned fish is also a very convenient and economical choice and has the same omega-3 benefits as fresh versions. I always have canned tuna, sardines, and salmon in my cupboard.

Once you choose your fish, you will be surprised how quick and easy it is to prepare deliciously. The simplest thing to do is brush a fish fillet with a little olive oil, add a little salt and pepper, and give it squeeze of lemon once it is done cooking. You can't go wrong simply baking it at 400°F for 8 to 10 minutes per every inch of thickness, or until it flakes easily with a fork. Broiling for that same amount of time works great for thin fillets. Grilling fish is also a cinch, but remember that flaky fish such as sole falls apart on the grill, so stick with a steaklike fish such as salmon or halibut or skewer up some shrimp or scallops, or pick up one of those handy grilling baskets.

action

Eat fish at least two times this week, choosing from the Usually or Sometimes list (see opposite).

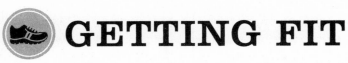
GETTING FIT

advanced strength training

This week you'll learn some new strength-building exercises you can add to your repertoire. I'll also describe some fun, easy ways to keep challenging your body with strength training.

PUMP IT UP In Week 6, I showed you how to make your walks more challenging by increasing their intensity. You can do the same thing with strength training.

Think of it this way. Say you do one set of 10 push-ups three times a week. The first couple of weeks, it feels difficult. Then, as your muscles get stronger and used to the demands being placed on them, it begins to get easier. That's good, and it means that you're growing stronger. But as the exercise becomes easier, it also means that your body isn't being challenged as much anymore. Eventually you'll hit a plateau and stop seeing results.

You started with one set of 8 to 12 reps of the strength-building moves. By this time, that's probably gotten pretty easy. To challenge yourself, you can add a set or two (so you're doing two or three sets of the basic moves), change the order in which you do them, or try different exercises. This week, I've included a series of new moves that work your legs first and then target your upper body. Start with one set of the moves and work up to two or three. Or you can try this workout one day a week and your original strength-training workout the other two days, or any combination you like. The key is to keep your muscles guessing.

advanced strengthening moves

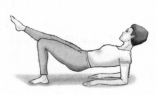

Lying hip raises (works muscles in the backs of the legs)
Lie on your back and raise yourself up on your elbows; your head and chest will be off the ground. Bend your left leg and place your left foot flat on the ground. Raise your extended right leg. Pushing down with your left heel and elbows, lift up your butt, squeezing your glutes and hamstrings, and slowly return to your original position with your butt on the ground. Do 8 to 12 reps before switching to the other leg.

Two-position push-up (works chest muscles and backs of upper arms) Assume a modified push-up position (lying flat,

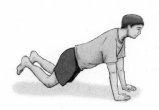

facing down, knees bent, weight on hands and knees) with both hands about six inches apart at breastbone level. Perform a push-up. When you return to the "up" position, move both hands (one at a time) so that they are slightly wider than shoulder width apart, and perform a push-up from this wide position. (If you're strong enough, you can do this move in a standard push-up position, keeping your weight on your hands and toes instead of hands and knees.) Then move back to the original position and repeat. Do 8 to 12 reps.

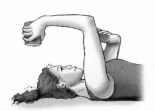

Superman (works back muscles) Lie facedown with your arms straight out over your head. While pointing your toes and reaching out as far as you can with your arms and legs, slowly raise both arms and legs off the floor. (Don't lift your head or look up.) Hold for three breaths and release slowly. Perform 8 to 12 reps.

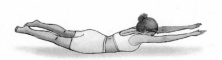

Supine single-arm extension (works muscles on the back of your arms) Lying faceup, hold a single dumbbell in your right hand and point your right arm straight up. Place two fingers of your left hand just below your right elbow, lightly touching your right triceps to help promote proper form. Keeping the upper arm still, slowly bend your right arm, letting the weight come down to your right shoulder before pressing it back up. Take three seconds to lower and three seconds to raise the weight. Perform 8 to 12 reps.

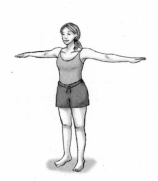

Sun gods (works shoulder muscles) Stand up and place your arms out to your sides at shoulder height, palms facing down. Keeping your arms straight and your fingers pointed out, make 50 small, quick circles toward the front of your body; then make 50 circles toward the rear of your body. Move your arms to shoulder height in front of your body, palms facing down, and make 50 of the same tight circles to the inside, then 50 to the outside. Finally, raise your arms above your head, palms facing in, and make 50 tight circles in one direction and 50 in the other.

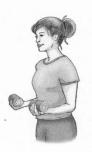

Controlled curls (works muscles in the front of your arms) Hold a dumbbell or can in each hand. Standing straight with arms at your sides, slowly bring your arms up halfway to your shoulders (your lower arms will be parallel to the ground) in a half-curl, counting up for four seconds and down for four seconds; do 7 reps. Then do 7 reps from the halfway point to your shoulders, again using a four-count. Finally, do 7 full curls using the four-count up and down. (This move breaks a normal curl up into two distinct sections to work your biceps, the muscles in the front of your upper arms, differently.)

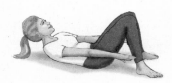

Laces (works stomach muscles) Lie on your back with your knees bent and feet flat on the floor, arms at your sides. Lift both shoulders off the floor with your chin up and, with your left hand, reach toward the front of your left foot (where your shoelaces would be); then return to your original position and reach toward your "laces" on your right foot with your right hand. Alternate for 25 reps on each side.

CIRCUIT TRAINING Circuit training has become increasingly popular. It combines cardiovascular activity with strength training, which makes it an effective way to burn calories and tone up at the same time—plus it's impossible to get bored because you're constantly switching activities. Yet you can significantly improve your cardiovascular fitness level by exercising in short bursts of approximately 60 seconds each.

Circuit training involves doing a "circuit" or series of strength-training exercises. Between each exercise, you jog, bike, jump rope, or otherwise stay active to keep your heart rate up, or you move immediately to the next exercise without resting. A circuit could be as simple as warming up, doing push-ups, jogging in place for a minute, doing lunges, jogging in place for another minute, doing squats, jogging in place for a minute, doing crunches, warming down, and then repeating the whole sequence once or twice.

The difficulty (and effectiveness) of a session depends on how many exercises you do, the speed and intensity at which you exercise, the length of intervals, the time you spend doing each exercise, and how many circuits you do. Basically, the greater the variety of activities, the better it is for overall fitness. Research shows that doing circuit training just once or twice a week can make a big difference in your fitness level. Give it a try to boost your regular routine.

Find Fitness Facts Online

Looking for fitness advice online? Check out these sites:

- **ACE Fitness "Fit Facts." www.acefitness.org/fitfacts**
Fit Facts, compiled by the American Council on Exercise, are one-page fact sheets that address a variety of health and fitness topics such as cardiovascular exercise, exercising with health challenges, and marathon and triathalon training.

- **About.com Exercise. www.exercise.about.com**
The "Exercise" section of About.com offers many tips and tricks on how to start exercising, how to get the most out of your workout, and the best music to listen to while exercising.

- **Fitness: Expert Answers, Mayo Clinic www.mayoclinic.com/health/fitness/MY00396/TAB=expertanswers**
Mayo Clinic's Fitness: Expert Answers page is a great resource if you need specific information or advice about topical exercise issues like the benefits of energy drinks, toning shoes, and whole body vibration, to name a few. All listed questions are answered by Mayo Clinic staff.

Circuit training should be challenging but not exhausting. Work at a comfortable pace for you—your goal is to keep your heart rate up during the cardio portions of the circuit, but you don't want to collapse after five minutes. You may find it easier to push yourself, though, because you know you're going to switch to a different activity after only a minute. It's a flexible way to train—if time is limited, circuit training can count as both cardio and strength training.

Before you circuit train, walk for five minutes to warm up. Have any equipment you'll need (weights, for example) handy. Decide in advance what order you'll perform the exercises in—for example, you can use the workout in this chapter or the original strength-training workout. Then, instead of resting in between exercises, jog or walk briskly in place to keep your heart rate up. At the end of the circuit, cool down and perform your stretching exercises.

OTHER WAYS TO PUMP IT UP Doing different exercises isn't the only way to give your body a new challenge. You can try these techniques, as well:

exercise myths debunked

Just as fad diets come and go, so do exercise trends. And much of the workout advice we hear through the grapevine has only a sliver of truth to it, if that. Here are some of the most common workout myths—and the facts behind them:

- **You burn more calories exercising on an empty stomach.** Not true—you expend the same number of calories during activity whether you've eaten or not. Exercising on an empty stomach can actually sabotage your workout if you run out of energy before you finish. A light snack that contains some carbohydrates and protein (see pages 84–85) about 90 minutes before you work out will give you energy to exercise. If you like to work out first thing in the morning, try something light like a cup of yogurt or half a banana.

- **Lifting weights bulks you up.** This may be a common fear among women, but it's unfounded. Women don't have as much testosterone as men do, so the average woman who weight trains will merely improve her overall muscle tone and look sleeker and firmer.

- **You must exercise for at least 30 minutes for health benefits.** Plenty of research shows that you can reap significant health benefits (think lowered blood pressure and lowered cholesterol) from as little as 10 minutes of moderate-intensity exercise like walking or doing yard work. In fact, new research reveals that the most significant health benefits occur in the first 5 minutes of activity you perform!

- **Crunches flatten your stomach.** Wrong! It seems like abdominal exercises would trim your tummy, but it doesn't work that way. "Spot reduction," or targeting one specific area of the body, will strengthen those muscles used but doesn't do much else. In other words, you can do thousands of crunches but you won't ever have a washboard stomach if there's a layer of fat on top of those muscles. The bottom line is that you can't selectively eliminate fat from particular parts of your body—you have to lose it all over by reducing your caloric intake and upping your activity.

- **You should stretch before you start your workout.** While this is a common myth, it's actually better to warm up a little *before* you stretch. The reason? Warm muscles stretch better, which reduces your chance of injury. For example, if you're going to walk, warm up for five minutes by strolling at an easy pace, and then stop and stretch before continuing your workout. Don't forget to perform some gentle, sustained stretches after exercise, as well, to help you maintain flexibility.

- **You'll burn more fat if you exercise at a slower pace.** This is a tricky one. Your body burns a mixture of fat and carbohydrates when you exercise. Working out at an easy pace, you'll burn a higher *percentage* of fat than if you exercise more intensely—but you'll also expend fewer *total* calories overall. So if you want to burn more calories while working out, up your intensity—you'll get more bang for your exercise buck, so to speak.

- **Morning is the best time to exercise.** For health benefits, it makes no difference whether you exercise in the morning, afternoon, or evening. While studies reveal that a.m. exercisers stick with it longer than those who work out later in the day, not everyone enjoys working out in the morning. The bottom line is to pick the time that works for you and that you can stick with. That's the best time for you.

Make it large. Want to target your muscles in a short amount of time? Give what weight lifters call "giant sets" a try. With a giant set, you do two or three exercises in a row that use the same muscles—like doing lunges and then immediately doing squats afterward. It's more difficult because you're increasing the amount of work your muscles have to perform.

Slow it down. Recently, "superslow" strength training has come into favor. It's always good to do strength-training moves in a slow, controlled fashion—it eliminates momentum and forces your muscles to work harder. Try slowing down your reps even more—take 10 seconds to lift and 10 seconds to return, for example. It's much more demanding.

Work to your max. Once your body gets stronger, you'll need to add more weights or more repetitions of an exercise to continue to challenge yourself. At the end of a set, your muscles should feel fatigued—if you feel like you could do another 5 or 10 reps, you're not working hard enough.

Hit the circuit. When you circuit train, you keep your heart rate high while doing different strength-training moves. It's a great way to add a cardiovascular component to your strength training.

action
Try the advanced strength-training workout, or experiment with circuit training.

 # FEELING GOOD

family ties

RECONNECTING WITH YOUR FAMILY The key to happiness for most people doesn't turn on fame, fortune, or even career success. While these things may play a part in overall satisfaction, it's relationships with the people we love that are likely to have the biggest influence on day-to-day satisfaction. Most of us realize that maintaining close relationships with those we love—especially our family—requires time and effort. Yet when time is in short supply, it's often our relationships, not our jobs or errands or even paying the bills, that suffer. We may schedule everything else in our lives, but we fail to make time for the people who are most important to us.

Take a minute to consider your relationships with your family members. Are your connections as close and meaningful as you would like them to be? Would you like to have more time to spend with those you love? Can you remember the last time you had a heart-to-heart talk with your children or spouse?

Think about ways you can reconnect. For example, it might be as simple as e-mailing your sister who lives out of state once a week, or planning a weekly no-TV family night to play games with your kids. What you do needn't be expensive or extravagant—there's simply no substitute for time with your family, especially your children. That doesn't mean you need to spend hours every day pondering the deepest questions of the universe with your teenager. You can have quality time during a trip to the grocery store or on the way home from school.

Connecting with kids. Chances are you ask your children the same question day after day: "How was school today?" Instead, ask something different: "What was the best thing that happened to you today?" "So, who's your favorite teacher right now? Why?" "What was the toughest thing you had to do today?" "If you could go anywhere, where would you go?" Ask questions and really *listen*. Set aside your natural urge to teach and help and protect. Don't try to correct your child. Just listen and connect.

Connecting with your partner. We often take our partners or spouses for granted, and most of our conversations with them revolve around basics—who will pick up the kids from the birthday party, when to replace the roof of the house, locating lost keys. You've already made a date with your child or children. Do the same with your partner. You don't have to make it an expensive evening out—the idea is that once a week you'll spend time together doing something fun and enjoying each other's company.

Connecting with your extended family. With your parents, siblings, and other relatives, decide that you'll make more of an effort. Take it beyond the standard "How are you?" and ask what's happening in their lives. Ask your parents and siblings to share memories with you. What are their hopes for the future? How are they spending their time? What's most important to them?

Social media have made it easier to stay connected with far-flung family members. If you want to stay in touch, consider different forms of communication and which works best for the person you're connecting with. Your mom may prefer an occasional phone call, while your nephew loves to text. It doesn't matter how you connect, just that you make the effort.

I've found Facebook and Twitter the fastest ways to keep up with both family and friends. In just a matter of minutes, I can admire photos of my girlfriend's new baby, check in with my sister-in-law, post my latest news. These sites do have an addictive quality; the average person spends about 15 hours per week online, and a quarter of that time is spent on social media sites likes Facebook and Twitter. It's become a part of everyday life for many people today.

There are no set rules for social media, so the way you use them will depend on you. I do have a few suggestions, though:

- Be mindful of what you post; remember that you never know who may see what you put online regardless of privacy settings. That goes for status updates, photos, videos, you name it.

- Be mindful of how you spend your time. Facebook games can be addicting, but is that really how you want to spend every evening?

- Use social media as an adjunct to your "real-life" relationships, not as a substitute for them. If you have five hundred friends on Facebook but haven't socialized with a friend in weeks, you may need to put more emphasis on face-to-face relationships.

Social media can help you build and strengthen your connections. They can help you stay close to your family and friends who live far away, but I don't think they will ever be a substitute for face-to-face relating—nothing can take the place of shared personal contact, conversations, and experiences.

action

Make a commitment to plan a special time with your partner or family. Do something fun—maybe something you haven't tried before, like going hiking or visiting the zoo or in-line skating in the park. Remember, this change is optional.

week 9 ACTION SUMMARY

 ### eating well

- Shop to replenish your healthy pantry.
- Eat regular meals and snacks, stopping when you are at 7 on the Hunger Continuum (see page 61).
- Drink enough to stay well hydrated, including at least five glasses of water and a maximum of one sugary drink a day.

- Use healthy fats for cooking, dressings, and spreads.
- Eat two to four servings of fruit and three to six servings of vegetables each day.
- Check the ingredient list on your food labels.
- Get at least three servings of whole grains a day and limit refined grains.
- Eat fish at least twice this week.
- Record in your journal everything you eat and drink.

getting fit

- Walk for 20 minutes three times at mid-intensity.
- Stretch and do strength training and core training three times.
- Include a fun element in your fitness program.
- Continue to attend a fitness class.
- Try advanced strengthening moves or circuit training.
- Note your activity in your journal.

feeling good

- Do the Five-Minute Breathing Exercise or take a minivacation once a day.
- Practice mindfulness.
- Say no to tasks you don't want to and don't have to do.
- Keep up your bedtime ritual.
- Do a deep relaxation or meditation exercise at least once.
- Optional:
  Tackle a clutter-clearing project.
  Explore journaling.
  Plan a special time with your partner or family.

WEIGHT

....

WEEK 10

this week's changes

1. Eat a serving of nuts, seeds, beans, or soy each day.

2. Increase the intensity of your walking.

3. Reconnect with a friend (optional).

this week's recipes

Full-Flavor Meatless Proteins

- Spiced Almonds
- Lentil Soup
- Stir-Fried Chinese Cabbage with Tofu
- White Chili
- Marinated Tofu
- Mixed Vegetables with Peanut Sauce

Each of these recipes is packed with hearty protein and big flavor, driving home the point that you don't need meat for dishes that are both filling and fulfilling. They will certainly make it easy for you to meet this week's goal of incorporating more nuts, seeds, and beans into your life.

spiced almonds

SERVES 8 *Seasoned almonds pack a whole lot of satisfaction, from their sweet-spicy-savory coating to their unbeatable crunch. They make an ideal afternoon snack. And almonds are not only tasty, they are one of the best sources of hard-to-get vitamin E.*

1 large egg white
2 teaspoons paprika
2 teaspoons dark brown sugar
¾ teaspoon salt
½ teaspoon Worcestershire sauce
¼ teaspoon cayenne pepper
2 cups natural almonds

1. Preheat the oven to 350°F. Line a baking sheet with parchment paper.

2. In a large bowl whisk together all the ingredients except the almonds until well combined. Add the almonds and toss until evenly coated. Transfer the almonds to the parchment-lined baking tray to form a single layer. Bake for 20 minutes, until the coating is crisp. Almonds will continue to crisp as they cool. Allow to cool completely, and then break up any nuts that are stuck together. Nuts will keep up to five days in an airtight container.

Calories 210; Fat 18 g (Sat 1.3 g, Mono 11 g, Poly 4.3 g); Protein 8 g; Carb 9 g; Fiber 4 g; Chol 0 mg; Sodium 230 mg

lentil soup

SERVES 8 TO 10 *I especially like lentils because they do not require presoaking and they are especially easy to digest. This hearty, belly-warming soup is a classic family favorite. Make a big pot of it on the weekend and freeze leftovers so that you have a healthy meal at the ready for busy weeknights.*

  2 tablespoons olive oil
  1 large onion, diced
  4 carrots, diced
  2 celery stalks, diced
  1 garlic clove, minced
  ¼ teaspoon dried thyme
  2 bay leaves
2½ cups lentils
 12 cups (two 48-ounce cans) low-sodium chicken broth
     or vegetable broth
  2 cups chopped fresh spinach, chard, or kale
  1 tablespoon balsamic vinegar
     Salt and freshly ground black pepper to taste

1. In a large soup pot, heat the oil over a medium-high flame. Add the onion, carrots, and celery, and cook until they begin to soften, about 3 minutes. Add the garlic and cook for 1 more minute. Stir in the thyme, bay leaves, and lentils. Add the broth and bring to a boil.

2. Simmer on low heat for 1 hour. Add the chopped greens and vinegar, and simmer for another 30 minutes. Season with salt and pepper to taste and serve.

Calories 325; Fat 7.1 g (Sat 2 g, Mono 3 g, Poly 1 g); Protein 23.9 g; Carb 44.5 g; Fiber 20.8 g; Chol 7.5 mg; Sodium 246 mg

stir-fried chinese cabbage with tofu

SERVES 4 *This stir-fry is superquick because there is not a lot of chopping to do, and it's especially flavorful, with loads of fresh ginger, garlic, and scallions. The tofu gives it a meaty heartiness. Serve over rice.*

3 small bunches bok choy (a type of Chinese cabbage, about 1 pound)
2 tablespoons canola oil
1 tablespoon peeled and grated fresh ginger
3 garlic cloves, minced
⅓ cup chopped scallion
1 pound marinated, cooked tofu, cut into cubes (see recipe on page 233) or use store-bought)
2 tablespoons low-sodium soy sauce
1 tablespoon sesame seeds

1. Cut 1 inch off the bottom of the bok choy and wash the separated stalks. Chop the bok choy crosswise into ½-inch-wide strips.

2. Heat the oil in a wok or large deep skillet over a medium flame. Add the ginger and garlic, and cook for 15 seconds, stirring constantly. Add the scallion and bok choy. Raise the heat to high and cook, stirring occasionally, for 5 minutes.

3. Stir in the marinated tofu, soy sauce, and ¼ cup water, and cook, stirring occasionally, until the liquid is reduced slightly and the tofu is warmed, about 2 minutes. Sprinkle with sesame seeds.

Calories 243; Fat 18.6 g (Sat 2.1 g, Mono 7.6 g, Poly 7.9 g); Protein 15.2 g; Carb 8.4 g; Fiber 2.4 g; Chol 0 mg; Sodium 688 mg

white chili

SERVES 6 *Chili is the perfect party food. Just keep a pot of it warm on the stove, put out the fixings, and let everyone help themselves.*

2 tablespoons olive oil
1 pound boneless chicken breast, cut into bite-size chunks
1 large onion, diced
3 garlic cloves, minced
2 (4-ounce) cans chopped mild green chilis, with juice
½ cup tomatillo salsa
1 (14.5-ounce) can low-sodium chicken broth
¼ teaspoon ground cumin
½ teaspoon dried oregano
2 (15.5-ounce) cans white beans, like cannellini, preferably low-sodium, drained and rinsed
3 tablespoons lime juice
Salt to taste
½ cup fresh cilantro, chopped
1 cup nonfat plain yogurt
½ cup shredded sharp cheddar cheese

1. Heat 1 tablespoon of the oil in a large saucepan over a medium-high flame. Add the chicken pieces and sauté for 5 minutes, or until cooked through. Remove from the pan and set aside.

2. Add the remaining tablespoon of oil and the onion to the pan, and sauté over medium heat until the onion is tender, about 3 minutes. Add the garlic and sauté for 1 minute more. Add the chilis, salsa, chicken broth, cumin, and oregano, and bring to a boil. Reduce the heat and simmer for 20 minutes.

3. Add the chicken and beans, and cook for 5 minutes more. Stir in the lime juice, then season with salt to taste. Serve topped with cilantro, yogurt, and cheese.

Calories 350; Fat 12 g (Sat 3.5 g, Mono 5.1 g, Poly 1.1 g); Protein 30 g; Carb 32 g; Fiber 8 g; Chol 60 mg; Sodium 540 mg

marinated tofu

SERVES 4 *Baked tofu is crispy on the outside, creamy inside, and loaded with flavor. Removing as much water as possible from the tofu before cooking it, as in this recipe, helps the tofu absorb the flavors of the marinade and cook up crisp rather than mushy. It is delicious eaten as is or in sandwiches, salads, or stir-fries. Serve hot or cold.*

1 pound extra-firm tofu
2 tablespoons low-sodium soy sauce
1 tablespoon orange juice
2 teaspoons sesame oil
1 teaspoon canola oil
Cooking spray

1. Slice the tofu into ½-inch-thick slabs and lay the slices on top of paper towels. Use more paper towels (you'll probably need three) and firmly pat the tofu in order to remove as much of the water as possible. Cut the tofu into ¾-inch cubes.

2. In a medium bowl, combine the soy sauce, orange juice, sesame oil, and canola oil. Add the tofu cubes and toss gently. Cover and let the tofu marinate in the refrigerator for at least 30 minutes, and up to 24 hours.

3. Preheat the oven to 450°F. Spray a large shallow baking dish with cooking spray. Place the tofu in a single layer in the baking dish. Bake for 25 to 30 minutes, or until golden brown.

Calories 145; Fat 10.4 g (Sat 1.4 g, Mono 3.1 g, Poly 5.3 g); Protein 12.3 g; Carb 3.4 g; Fiber .5 g; Chol 0 mg; Sodium 311 mg

mixed vegetables with peanut sauce

SERVES 4 *This rich, satisfying meal gets its protein from peanuts. Serve over rice.*

   1 teaspoon canola oil
   1 large garlic clove, minced
   ½ cup natural-style creamy peanut butter
   ⅛ teaspoon cayenne pepper
   1 tablespoon cider vinegar or white wine vinegar
   1 tablespoon honey
   2 tablespoons low-sodium soy sauce
   ¼ teaspoon salt
   3 cups whole string beans, strings removed and ends cut off
   4 large carrots, cut on the diagonal into thin rounds
   1 large head broccoli, cut into spears
   1 teaspoon toasted sesame oil
   ½ cup chopped scallions

1. Heat the canola oil in a medium saucepan over a medium flame. Reduce the heat to low, add the garlic, and sauté until fragrant, about 1 minute. Stir in the peanut butter, cayenne pepper, vinegar, honey, soy sauce, salt, and 1½ cups water, mixing thoroughly. The mixture will become creamy as it heats up and with additional stirring. Simmer on the lowest possible heat for 30 minutes, stirring occasionally.

2. Meanwhile, steam the string beans, carrots, and broccoli in a large steamer for about 15 minutes, or until tender.

3. Arrange the cooked vegetables on a plate and top with the peanut sauce. Drizzle with sesame oil and garnish with scallions.

Calories 336; Fat 19.4 g (Sat 3.7 g, Mono 8.9 g, Poly 5.6 g); Protein 16 g; Carb 33.6 g; Fiber 12 g; Chol 0 mg; Sodium 669 mg

EATING WELL

a new food group: nuts, seeds, and legumes

There's nothing like the fun of shelling and eating peanuts at a ball game, ladling up some hearty bean chili on a cold winter's day, or sprinkling your favorite nuts to spice up an otherwise dull salad. Think these can be only occasional indulgences? Nope—they're treats you don't have to feel guilty about. Nuts, seeds, and legumes (beans, lentils, dried peas, peanuts, and soy) are incredibly healthy and can help you keep your weight in check. This week we're going to get a little nutty (and "beany") as we explore ways to get more of these delicious nuggets into your life.

Because they are great sources of protein, nuts, seeds, and legumes have traditionally been lumped as a "meat alternative" into the same basic food group as meat. But emerging science reveals that these protein-packed plants offer so many unique health benefits that they should be much more than meat's understudy—in fact, they should be on the main stage. These vegetable proteins are so important, I believe they deserve a food group of their very own, so I have given them one in the Small Changes, Big Results eating plan.

I am not the first to grant nuts, seeds, and legumes their own food group. The folks at the National Institutes of Health did it when they created their DASH (Dietary Approaches to Stop Hypertension) Diet. Studies proved that this eating plan dramatically reduced blood pressure in only two weeks! The DASH diet is similar to the one I'm discussing here: a plan that is rich in fruits, vegetables, whole grains, low-fat dairy products, lean meats, poultry, fish, and the headliner of this week's chapter, a new sixth food group: nuts, seeds, and legumes.

There are reams of evidence supporting the health benefits of these wonderful foods. As a whole, they are all great sources of protein, fiber, potassium, zinc, and magnesium. Individually, they each have different properties that protect your health and expand your mealtime options.

GO A LITTLE NUTS (AND SEEDS) Nuts used to be considered a sinful treat, high in fat and calories—a food nibbled guiltily in a bar or at holiday parties. Well, you can erase any notion of nuts as a no-no, because nuts (including tree nuts like almonds, walnuts, pecans, and hazelnuts, as well as peanuts, which are a nutlike legume), nut butters, and seeds are just plain good for you.

Check this out: nuts are loaded with healthy monounsaturated fat, which has been shown to lower bad cholesterol and help keep blood sugar steady. (Flaxseeds and walnuts also contain hard-to-get omega-3 fats.) Nuts are chock-full of important nutrients like vitamin E, magnesium, calcium, zinc, copper, iron, and of course protein. Plus they are packed with protective phytochemicals and fiber. There is so much evidence that eating nuts reduces the risk of heart disease, the Food and Drug Administration even lets nut packagers boast about it on their labels.

Because they are such a satisfying food, nuts and seeds can also help you manage your weight. A small handful of nuts and a piece of fruit can help you get past those afternoon cravings for sweets and give you the stamina you need to get in some exercise or make it through the rest of your day. They're also an ideal on-the-go snack to stash in your bag or desk drawer until hunger calls.

One thing, though: notice I said a *small* handful. Nuts, nut butters, and seeds are high in calories, so if you suddenly start eating piles of nuts or scoops of peanut butter out of the jar in addition to what you are already consuming, you will probably gain weight. The trick is to substitute a small portion of nuts—say, about ⅓ cup nuts, ¼ cup seeds, or 2 tablespoons of nut butter—*instead* of less healthy options. Grab a handful of almonds and a piece of fruit instead of a candy bar or chips in the afternoon. Spread some peanut butter on your toast in the morning in lieu of butter or cream cheese. Or toss some pumpkin seeds on your salad at lunch instead of bacon bits or cheese, both of which are high in saturated fat.

COOL BEANS The variety of dishes that start with the simple little bean is astounding. Nearly every culture around the world boasts a delicious and unique bean dish. Think about it—there are red beans and rice in Latin and Caribbean cultures; dahl, an Indian lentil stew; Middle Eastern hummus (pureed chickpeas and sesame paste); black-eyed peas and rice in the West Indies; Italian *pasta e fagioli* (pasta and white beans); and edamame (young green soybeans) in Japan. Some North American favorites include baked beans, hopping john (black-eyed peas), and traditional bean chili. Then there are the soups—lentil, split pea, white bean and garlic, navy bean, minestrone. The list goes on. If you think eating healthfully has to be boring or you yawn just thinking about another plain chicken breast, wake up to any of these exciting bean dishes.

People have gotten so creative with beans and other legumes like dried peas and lentils because they have all been a dietary staple for centuries. They're inexpensive and easy to prepare yet provide essential protein, B vitamins, zinc, copper, magnesium, iron, potassium, fiber, and antioxidants. They are also one of the best sources of folate, the B vitamin we now know prevents birth defects and guards against heart disease. One cup of beans provides almost a full day's worth of folate! Plus beans have virtually no fat, and they are incredibly satisfying, which means you can feel comfortably full eating beans without packing on calories.

Beans are sometimes shunned as a poor man's food, providing cheap protein for those who can't afford meat. But thanks to the bean's incredible nutrient profile, people who get more of their protein from beans, and less from fatty meats, will find they are much richer health-wise.

So next time you crave Mexican food, skip the beef tacos and go for the bean burrito instead. Try a filling, fragrant bowl of split pea or lentil soup for lunch, or sprinkle some garbanzo beans, also known as chickpeas, on your salad. Premade hummus is a staple in my fridge. It makes for an excellent lunch on the run. Just spread some on a whole wheat pita, stuff in some prewashed greens, and you've got a portable, filling sandwich.

While it's easy to prepare dried beans, they do take time. Dried beans need to be soaked overnight and then cooked for one to four hours. I usually don't think that far ahead, so I keep a variety of canned beans at my fingertips. Yes, canned beans can be fairly high in salt, whereas dried beans have almost none. But rinsing canned beans under cold water gets rid of about a third of the sodium, and low-sodium canned beans are now widely available. You simply can't beat the convenience. Some quick meal ideas: toss a can of white beans into your pasta sauce while it is heating; sauté chopped onion, garlic, and green peppers, add a can of black beans, and serve over rice; or substitute half the meat in your favorite beef chili recipe with red beans (use one 15-ounce can of beans per pound of meat).

I know you're thinking it, so let's be frank. You say you avoid beans because they give you gas? Well, there are ways to minimize this uncomfortable side effect (or should I say sound effect?). First, if you haven't had beans in a while, don't dig into a big bean-laden bowl of chili just yet. Start with a small bowl. You want to introduce beans into your diet gradually, so that your body has a chance to adapt.

If you use dried beans, draining and rinsing them after soaking eliminates some of the gas-causing compounds. Cooking your beans thoroughly also helps. Canned beans are usually already well cooked; rinsing them before you prepare them eliminates a lot of the "gas factor."

Once you have built up your tolerance, enjoy beans regularly. You're less likely to suffer from gas when your body is used to these fiber-rich foods.

BEYOND TOFU Soybeans are legumes like those I've been talking about. But soy has such unique properties that it is often considered in a class all its own. In recent years, soy has become increasingly popular, and there are now dozens of soy-based foods, including tofu, soy milk, tempeh (a savory fermented soybean cake), soy nuts, soy cheese, and miso (a rich fermented soybean paste used for flavoring and as a soup base). Now you can even buy soy burgers, soy hot dogs, soy "chicken" nuggets, and, believe it or not, soy bacon.

Soy has been making big headlines. First it was hyped as a miracle food, and then decried as potentially dangerous. What's the bottom line? First, soy has numerous benefits. It has been shown to reduce cholesterol, fight certain cancers, and help prevent osteoporosis; it also may alleviate the symptoms of menopause in some women. And according to the FDA, 25 grams of soy protein a day (about four servings' worth of tofu or soybeans) has been shown to reduce the risk of heart disease.

When eaten in excess, soy may have negative effects for some people. If you have a history of breast cancer, thyroid problems, or kidney stones, ask your doctor whether you should limit the amount of soy you eat. Many processed soy foods, like protein bars and powders, have a very high concentration of soy protein, making it easier to consume more than is healthy. I recommend avoiding highly processed soy foods and eating tofu, edamame, miso, and soy milk. A daily serving or two of the latter is a healthy addition to most people's diets.

Soy is chock-full of nutrients like B vitamins, minerals, fiber, and healthy fats. But soy's benefits are mainly attributed to the type of protein it contains, along with a powerful group of compounds called isoflavones. Different soy foods have varying amounts of naturally occurring protein and isoflavones. Soy flour, soy nuts, soybeans, soy milk, tempeh, and tofu are among the best sources. While soy can be good for you, cooking—and eating—soy can be intimidating. Many people assume they won't like it or don't know how to cook it. There are plenty of user-friendly, tasty soy foods out there. Simply grill up a delicious soy burger just as you would a beef burger. Soy milk is delicious in a shake or on cereal. Soy nuts are a crunchy and flavorful snack on their own and make a great salad topping, as well.

That white, tasteless block of tofu may make you run away in fear. But tofu takes on the flavors of marinades beautifully and is easy to prepare. (See Marinated Tofu, page 233.) And to make life even easier, many stores now carry premarinated, precooked tofu that you can simply cut up for salads, stir-fries, or casseroles.

Finally, there is one of my favorite soy foods, edamame (young green soybeans), found either in the pod or shelled. They are often sold frozen and are perfect to have on hand at home—to prepare them, simply boil them for about five minutes. Served in the pod, they are a wonderful healthy finger food. Just work the beans out of the pod with your teeth, eat the beans, and discard the empty pod. Use shelled edamame just as you would any other bean, in salads, stews, and soups. With all these easy options, there is no reason not to give soy a try.

action

Include at least one serving of nuts, beans, seeds, or soy in your diet each day. One serving is ½ cup cooked beans or tofu, 1 cup soy milk, ⅓ cup nuts, ¼ cup seeds, or 2 tablespoons nut butter.

for vegetarians (and those who love them)

Susanne was worried when her 12-year-old came home from school and announced that she was no longer going to eat meat. "I'm a vegetarian now," Sasha declared. "No more animals for me."

After doing some research on a healthy vegetarian diet, Susanne realized that it wouldn't be that difficult to help her daughter meet her protein needs. By adding more meatless meals into her family's repertoire and making sure that Sasha still ate a balanced diet—even excluding animals—Susanne was confident that her Sasha was getting the nutrition she needed. Now in college, Sasha is still a committed vegetarian—and just as healthy as her two older, meat-eating brothers.

If you are a vegetarian (or someone you love is), you'll want to pay special attention to the foods highlighted this week—nuts, seeds, beans, and soy. They are often the protein mainstays of the vegetarian's diet.

While animal sources of protein contain all of the essential amino acids our bodies need, no single plant source can provide all the essential amino acids in quantities we need. However, certain foods "complement" one another to offer complete protein—in other words, eating both types of foods provides your body with all of the essential amino acids it needs. Nuts, seeds, beans, and soy are rich in the amino acids (protein's building blocks) that grains lack, and vice versa. Most vegetarians I know get plenty of grains but fall woefully short in the nut, seed, and bean category. It is critical to have both complementary groups in your diet each day, although you don't need to consume them at the same meal, as was once thought.

Are you thinking that if you eat cheese and milk, you needn't worry about consuming beans? Wrong. While milk products offer a complete protein and provide lots of calcium and vitamin D, they are poor sources of zinc and iron, minerals that many vegetarians don't get enough of. Nuts, seeds, beans, and soy are excellent sources of these essential minerals. So whether you are a vegan (someone who eats no animal products) or a lacto-ovo vegetarian (someone who eats no meat, fish, or poultry but consumes eggs and dairy products), you need to get at least two or three servings from the nuts, seeds, beans, and soy group every day.

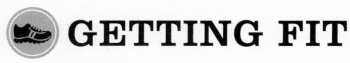

GETTING FIT

walking to the max

You've been walking regularly for more than two months now and have learned how to increase your intensity from low to medium. This week, you'll learn how to ratchet up to high intensity.

A few weeks ago, I explained how to take your cardiovascular exercise up a notch and make it more intense. You'll recall that you can do this by increasing the amount of time you exercise, the intensity at which you exercise, or the grade you're walking on (it's more difficult walking up a steep slope than a flat surface).

Most people are comfortable doing low- to moderate-intensity exercise; it's challenging but not too difficult. Once your body has become accustomed to moderate-intensity exercise, however, you can reap even more benefits by adding some high-intensity sessions to your workout program.

High-intensity exercise burns more calories per minute than low- or moderate-intensity exercise because you're placing more demands on your cardiovascular system and your muscles. Your body must work harder, so you burn more calories. High-intensity exercise also elevates your metabolism more than a moderate-intensity workout and has a greater "afterburn effect," meaning that your body burns even more calories after exercise than it would normally.

Competitive athletes and other highly trained exercisers may do high intensity two or three times a week; however, for most people, one or two high-intensity sessions a week is more than enough. Again, if you're exercising three times a week at moderate intensity, that's great. If you're ready to take it up a notch, choose one of these options:

- Walk for 40 minutes at mid-intensity; or

- Walk for 30 minutes, including some "intervals," or bursts, where you walk as fast as you can (that makes it high-intensity exercise); or

- Walk for 30 minutes with hills; or

- Walk and run for 30 minutes.

INTERVAL TRAINING Doing intervals will make your workouts more challenging, and you'll burn additional calories and improve your overall fitness in the process. When you do intervals, you purposely increase your intensity for short bursts of time, interspersing those bursts with rest or recovery periods. By doing so, your body is forced to work much harder than it's used to, and that's the whole point.

While athletes use intervals to drop their times and win competitions, interval training pays benefits to even everyday exercisers. First, it forces you to use your fast-twitch muscle fibers, which may not be used during low- or moderate-intensity exercise. (Your muscles contain both "fast-twitch" and "slow-twitch" fibers, which are recruited depending on what type of activity you do. Long, slow, aerobic exercise usually depends on slow-twitch fibers, while more intense exercise relies on fast-twitch fibers.) Second, interval training helps make your heart stronger and improves your ability to use oxygen efficiently.

Interval training also burns calories at a faster rate than exercising at a slower pace. If you intersperse a few intervals throughout your normal cardio work, you'll burn more calories during the exercise itself as well as afterward, due to the "afterburner" effect.

Raise Your Walking Ante

Uninspired by your usual walking route? Check out www.mapmy walk.com. This site includes 15 million different walking routes, so you can search for one near your home or workplace. Go online, pick a route, and go! Or create your own walking routes, measure them, and then keep track of how low long it takes you to complete them. You may find that you push yourself harder to beat your own "personal record."

Ready to try some interval training of your own? You can do intervals during your regular cardio workout, whether it's walking, jogging, cycling, rowing, or climbing stairs. All you need is a watch to track the interval times.

As with any cardio workout, warm up first. You may also want to do some stretches, after you warm up but before you begin the intervals. Remember that you're going to be working harder than normal and recruiting fast-twitch muscles, so you may feel out of breath and your muscles may "burn" a little.

A 1:1 ratio is usually a good place to begin. For example, you might walk slowly for five minutes to warm up, and then walk as fast as you can for one minute, then walk slowly for one minute, and repeat five times; then finish the workout at your usual pace to cool down.

As you get fitter, you can extend the effort times. Try a 2:1 ratio, for example—walk fast for two minutes, then slowly for one minute. Or you may want to do your usual workout for 20 minutes or so and then add intervals at the end (they can be tiring).

READY TO RUN? Many walkers are happy continuing to walk for fitness. They make their walks more challenging by increasing their speed or distance, or adding hills or inclines to work harder. Others get bitten by the running bug and decide they'd like to try jogging or running instead.

Running is a more demanding physical activity than walking, but at this point, you should be ready for a new challenge. Start by walking to warm up. After 5 or 10 minutes, begin to run slowly for a minute or so; then walk for a minute or until you catch your breath. Run again for a minute, then walk a minute. Maintain this routine for 30 minutes.

When you run, your head should be up, your chest lifted, arms relaxed at your sides. Don't let your head and shoulders hang forward as you tire; maintain proper posture as you run. You should be running heel to toe (that is, your heel strikes the ground first, then you roll onto your toes to push off), and your steps should be light. If you're slapping the ground, make an effort to run "lighter."

Depending on how you feel, you can increase your sessions from 1:1 (running 1 minute, walking 1 minute) to 2:1 (running 2 minutes, walking 1 minute) and so on as you become fitter. Work up to 20 to 30 minutes of easy running over time.

READY, SET, HIKE! Hiking is another way to boost the intensity of your regular walks. Hiking or trail walking is usually more challenging than walking because you're covering rougher, often hilly terrain. Hiking forces you to work harder because you're negotiating inclines and rougher footing than you may be used to. The faster you walk, the tougher it gets, but you can also choose to simply stroll. Either way, you'll be targeting the major muscles in your legs—your quadriceps, hamstrings, calves, and glutes.

The real beauty of hiking, though, is that it gives you a chance to slow down and reconnect with nature while you move your body. Finding a place to hike is often easier than you might think. Local, state, and national parks are all good places. Some have maps and marked trails; some do not. If you're new to hiking, stick to shorter, well-marked trails. With elevation changes, you may find a two-mile hike more challenging than a three-mile walk on a flat surface.

While you can usually wear your walking clothes for hiking, bring a jacket or other outer layer in case it gets chilly—the weather can change quickly, especially if you're hiking at higher altitudes. The same rules about layering clothes when you walk (see Keeping Warm in Cold Weather, page 47) apply: start with a T-shirt or tank top if the weather's warm, but take along an extra layer or two. You may also want to wear hiking shoes or boots, which are designed to give better traction on slippery trails or rough terrain. Their thick soles will also protect your feet from rocks and other objects on the trail.

Depending on how long your hike will be, you'll also want to take along a backpack or fanny pack. Plan to take more food and more water than you think you'll need—it's better to be overprepared than underprepared. Bring easily portable food like trail mix, energy bars, or fruit, a plastic bag for garbage, a flashlight, a map, and a compass if you'll be walking on unmarked trails. A simple first-aid kit that contains an Ace bandage, Band-Aids, antiseptic spray, and a cell phone for emergencies is also a good idea.

Finally, check the weather forecast before you go. A little rain won't hurt you, but you don't want to be hiking in an electrical storm or other severe weather.

CHECK OUT CROSS-TRAINING Do any activity day in, day out, and you're bound to get bored. Cross-training can help prevent that. When you cross-train, you perform other types of exercise in addition to or instead of your usual one. It helps prevent burnout, reduces your risk of injuries, and constantly challenges your body, which means you get more results from your program.

To cross-train, choose an activity that uses different muscle groups, or uses the same muscle groups in different ways. For example, walking is a great overall exercise, but biking puts a bigger demand on your glutes (butt muscles), quadriceps (the muscles in the fronts of your thighs), and calves as well as your arms, shoulders, and back. Swimming and rowing, on the other hand, use more of the muscles in your upper body than walking does.

Even if you have a favorite cardio activity, do something different at least one day a week. You might use a stair climber instead of a stationary bike, or try the elliptical trainer instead of using the treadmill like you usually do.

Focusing on what you're doing means you're more likely to get into a flow state, where you're only thinking of what you're doing, and that's a great mental and physical release.

action

This week, do at least one of your three walks at high intensity by increasing your walking speed and time, or adding more hills or inclines to your walk. If you like, you can choose to go hiking instead.

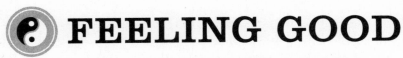

FEELING GOOD

reconnecting with friends

Last week, I talked about the importance of maintaining close relationships with family members. This week, I want you to think about the relationships you have with the other people in your life—your friends, coworkers, neighbors, and others you have daily contact with. Who do you consider your friends? Would you like closer relationships with them, or to spend more time with them?

Research shows that friendships not only enhance your life but also protect and improve your health. And studies show that the happiest people are those who have both good mental health and good social relationships.

Some people have one or two close friends and a large circle of acquaintances; others have an extended group of people they're close to. Over time, new friendships are made through circumstance or shared interests, while others are lost. It's natural to put our jobs and families ahead of our friends, but making time for people who you connect with and can laugh and share your life with only enriches your life.

Friendships take time and tending the same way your relationships with your family do. Keeping in touch—whether it's with phone calls, texts, Tweets, or e-mails—can nurture bonds whether you live across town or across the country. Make time for actual "face time," too, when you can; there's no substitute for the company of someone you love and truly enjoy.

OUTGROWING A FRIEND It may be that the two of you used to be close and now feel that you don't have much in common anymore. Or perhaps things have happened that make you feel as though the friendship isn't worth your time. Think about your relationship with the person. Does she support you, believe in you, have your best interests in mind? Do you enjoy talking to her and spending time with her? Everyone has down days, but if you're sapped by speaking to her for even a few minutes, it may be time to end the relationship. (I call these people energy vampires because they're so good at draining you!) You can simply stop calling or e-mailing. He or she will get the message. Remember, too, that ending a relationship that isn't good for you anymore makes more time in your life for people who will bring you joy and pleasure.

If this is a relationship that's really important to you, you may want to talk to your friend about the problem before you end it. Tell her how you feel and ask if there's a way to reconnect. Maybe there's something going on in her life that has affected her—something you don't know about. You won't know unless you ask.

ABOUT FORGIVENESS To err is human, to forgive divine, as the saying goes. Forgiving someone when he or she has hurt you can be extremely difficult. But true forgiveness can set the stage for a deeper relationship, help prevent disagreements about inconsequential things, and improve your own health. Studies show that forgiveness is good for the heart as well as the soul. Harboring a grudge or resentment against someone or something can only have a negative effect on your health. Forgiving someone can release this negative energy and have a positive impact on how you feel.

Many people find that writing a letter to the person who hurt them is helpful. Get out all your feelings and frustrations on paper. Pretend you're in front of the person and this is your chance to tell them everything. Then rip the letter into tiny pieces or burn it. (Or, try talking to someone close to you about what happened to let you vent and gain perspective.)

Then make a conscious effort to let it go—after you've forgiven someone, don't keep bringing up the same incident. Dwelling on it, especially with the other person, may prevent you from really forgiving.

action

This week, if you like, make an effort to reconnect with someone you're close to but haven't spoken to in a while.

week 10 ACTION SUMMARY

 eating well

- Shop to replenish your healthy pantry.
- Eat regular meals and snacks, stopping when you are at 7 on the Hunger Continuum (see page 61).
- Drink enough to stay well hydrated, including at least five glasses of water and a maximum of one sugary drink a day.
- Use healthy fats for cooking, dressings, and spreads.
- Eat two to four servings of fruit and three to six servings of vegetables each day.

continues ›››

- Check the ingredient list on your food labels.
- Get at least three servings of whole grains a day and limit refined grains.
- Eat fish at least twice this week.
- Eat at least one serving of nuts, seeds, beans, or soy each day.
- Record in your journal everything you eat and drink.

 ## getting fit

- Walk for 20 to 40 minutes three times at mid- or high intensity.
- Stretch and do strength training and core training three times.
- Include a fun element in your fitness program.
- Continue to attend a fitness class.
- Note your activity in your journal.

feeling good

- Do the Five-Minute Breathing Exercise or take a minivacation once a day.
- Practice mindfulness.
- Say no to tasks you don't want to and don't have to do.
- Keep up your bedtime ritual.
- Do a deep relaxation or meditation exercise at least once.
- Optional:
  Tackle a clutter-clearing project.
  Continue journaling.
  Plan a special time with your partner or family.
  Reconnect with a friend.

WEIGHT

....

WEEK

11

this week's changes

1. Switch to lean meats.

2. Increase the physical activity in your everyday life.

3. Do something to pamper your body (optional).

this week's recipes

Lean and Luscious Meat Dishes

- Roast Pork Tenderloin
- Venison with Mushroom-Wine Sauce
- Sesame Beef with Broccoli
- Beefsteak Soft Tacos
- Paprika-Rubbed Turkey Breast
- Chipotle Turkey Meat Loaf

You don't need to give up meat to eat healthy, you just have to do it right. That means keeping it lean and making portions smart-sized. These meat dishes are designed to punch up the flavor of lean meat and amp up sensible servings so that they are truly sumptuous and filling.

roast pork tenderloin

SERVES 4 *Whip up this easy marinade, add the pork tenderloins, and pop in the fridge before you head out for the day. When you return for the dinner rush, you will have a juicy, flavorful roast pork main course on the table, effortlessly, in about 15 minutes.*

2 tablespoons low-sodium soy sauce
2 tablespoons canola oil
2 tablespoons orange juice
1 garlic clove, minced
1 teaspoon peeled and freshly grated ginger, or ½ teaspoon ground ginger
1 teaspoon freshly ground black pepper
2 pork tenderloins (about ¾ pound each)

1. In a large bowl, whisk together the soy sauce, oil, orange juice, garlic, ginger, and pepper. Add the tenderloins, cover, and let marinate in the refrigerator for 2 to 8 hours. Preheat the broiler.

2. Place the pork in a roasting pan and broil for 15 minutes, 2 to 4 inches from the flame, turning the meat once at the halfway point.

Calories 250; Fat 11 g (Sat 1.5 g, Mono 5.7 g, Poly 2.6 g); Protein 36 g; Carb 1 g; Fiber 0 g; Chol 90 mg; Sodium 360 mg

venison with mushroom-wine sauce

SERVES 4 *Earthy mushrooms, wine, and tomato bring out the best in this tender game meat. The mushrooms, with their meaty texture, round out the portion, so you get an extra-generous amount on your plate. If you can't get venison, pork tenderloin works well, too.*

⅓ cup all-purpose flour
¼ teaspoon salt, plus more to taste
¼ teaspoon freshly ground black pepper, plus more to taste
1 to 1½ pounds boneless venison steak, cut into ½-inch-thick slices
1 tablespoon olive oil
¼ cup chopped shallots
1 garlic clove, minced
1½ cups chopped mushrooms
1 tablespoon tomato paste
½ cup red wine
½ cup low-sodium chicken broth

1. Mix the flour, salt, and pepper in a shallow dish. Dredge the meat in the seasoned flour. Heat the oil in a large skillet over medium-high. Cook the venison for 2 minutes per side, and then transfer to a plate and cover to keep warm.

2. Reduce the heat in the skillet to medium, add the shallots and garlic, and cook for 1 minute, stirring constantly. Add the mushrooms and sauté for about 3 minutes. Stir in the tomato paste. Add the wine and chicken broth, raise heat to medium-high, and cook for 1 minute more. Return the meat to the pan and simmer until heated, about 1 minute. Season with salt and pepper to taste.

Calories 276; Fat 7.8 g (Sat 2 g, Mono 3.5 g, Poly 1.3 g); Protein 35.5 g; Carb 10.4 g; Fiber .6 g; Chol 121 mg; Sodium 272 mg

sesame beef
with broccoli

SERVES 4 *Slicing meat thin and serving it with loads of veggies make a smart portion of beef seem luxuriously plentiful. That's one reason—in addition to the big, bold flavors—why stir-fries like this are so satisfying.*

- 1 pound top round or flank steak, thinly sliced against the grain
- ⅛ teaspoon salt
- 2 tablespoons canola oil, divided
- 1 small onion, sliced into half-moons
- 1 red bell pepper, seeded and thinly sliced
- 3 garlic cloves, thinly sliced
- 2 teaspoons minced fresh ginger
- 1 cup low-sodium beef broth
- 3 tablespoons low-sodium soy sauce
- 1 tablespoon honey
- ¼ teaspoon chili flakes
- 2 teaspoons cornstarch dissolved in 2 tablespoons cold water
- 1 large head of broccoli, cut into 1-inch florets (about 5 cups)
- 2 teaspoons toasted sesame oil
- 1 tablespoon sesame seeds, toasted in a dry skillet over a medium-high heat, stirring frequently, until golden brown, 2 minutes

1. Season the meat with salt. Heat 2 teaspoons of the oil in a large, deep skillet or wok that has a cover over a medium-high heat. Add half the beef and cook, stirring once or twice, until it is browned and just cooked through, about 5 minutes. Using a slotted spoon, transfer the meat to a plate and cover to keep warm. Add 2 more teaspoons of oil to the pan and repeat with the remaining beef.

2. Add the remaining 2 teaspoons of oil to the pan. Add the onion and pepper, and cook until slightly softened, about 2 minutes. Add the garlic and ginger, and cook an additional 30 seconds.

3. In a small bowl whisk together the beef broth, soy sauce, honey, and chili flakes, and add to the pan. Stir in the dissolved cornstarch and stir until the mixture comes to a boil. Stir in the broccoli, reduce the heat to medium-low, cover, and cook, stirring occasionally, until the broccoli is just tender and the liquid has thickened, about 5 minutes.

4. Add the beef back to the pan and stir to combine. Drizzle with sesame oil and sprinkle with sesame seeds.

Calories 290; Fat 15 g (Sat 2.5 g, Mono 7.1 g, Poly 3.7 g); Protein 29 g; Carb 15 g; Fiber 3 g; Chol 50 mg; Sodium 460 mg

beefsteak soft tacos

SERVES 4 *Soft corn tortillas, lean beef, and crunchy cabbage make these tacos especially healthy and make a sensible portion of meat go a long, satisfying way. They are a breeze to make and fun to eat.*

½ cup freshly squeezed lime juice
3 garlic cloves, minced
2 teaspoons chili powder
1 tablespoon olive oil
1¼ pounds top sirloin steaks
12 small corn tortillas (5 to 6 inches in diameter)
¾ cup store-bought tomato salsa
4 cups shredded cabbage
½ cup chopped cilantro
½ cup chopped scallions

1. In a large bowl, whisk together ¼ cup of the lime juice with the garlic, chili powder, and oil. Put the steaks in the bowl, turn them to distribute the marinade, cover, and marinate in the refrigerator for 1 hour.

2. Remove the steaks from the marinade and discard the marinade. Grill the steaks over medium heat for about 12 minutes for medium-rare, turning once. Carve into thin slices.

3. Place the tortillas on the grill to warm, turning once, about 30 seconds.

4. To prepare the tacos, place a few slices of meat on a warm tortilla, top with a tablespoon of salsa, ⅓ cup shredded cabbage, 2 teaspoons cilantro, 2 teaspoons scallions, and 1 teaspoon lime juice. Serve open-faced, so the diner can fold it, or fold and secure with a toothpick before serving.

Calories 426; Fat 10.3 g (Sat 3 g, Mono 4.5 g, Poly 14 g); Protein 40 g; Carb 44.4 g; Fiber 6.7 g; Chol 82 mg; Sodium 324 mg

paprika-rubbed turkey breast

SERVES 6 *Why reserve fresh turkey for holidays? This spice-rubbed roasted breast is a cinch to make, and the leftovers make terrific sandwiches the next day.*

½ boneless turkey breast (about 2 pounds), skin removed
2 teaspoons olive oil
1 teaspoon paprika
½ teaspoon garlic powder
½ teaspoon salt
¼ teaspoon freshly ground black pepper

1. Preheat the oven to 375°F. Rinse the turkey breast, pat dry, and put into a 9 × 11-inch baking dish.

2. In a small bowl combine the oil, paprika, garlic powder, salt, and pepper, and rub the mixture into the turkey breast.

3. Cook until the juices run clear when pierced with a fork and an instant-read meat thermometer inserted into the thickest part of the turkey registers 165°F, about 40 minutes. Let rest, covered with foil, for 10 minutes before slicing into ¼-inch slices.

Calories 180; Fat 2.5 g (Sat .5 g, Mono 1.27 g, Poly .45 g); Protein 37 g; Carb 0 g; Fiber 0 g; Cholesterol 95 mg; Sodium 270 mg

chipotle turkey meat loaf

SERVES 8 *I am always tickled that I manage to sneak a whole grain (oats) and a vegetable (zucchini) into this full-flavored meat loaf. Besides being healthy additions, they help the dish earn its reputation as the moistest meat loaf ever. The chipotle chili powder gives it the perfect tongue-tingling warmth, but if you prefer it more mild, you can use regular chili powder instead.*

Cooking spray
1 tablespoon canola oil
1 medium onion, finely chopped
½ green bell pepper, finely chopped
3 garlic cloves, minced
2 teaspoons ground cumin
2 teaspoons chipotle chili powder, or other chili powder
1 teaspoon ground coriander
1 teaspoon dried oregano
¾ teaspoon salt
2 pounds lean ground turkey
1 small zucchini (6 ounces), shredded (1¼ cups)
2 large eggs, lightly beaten
¾ cup quick-cooking oats
1 (8-ounce) can no-salt-added tomato sauce

1. Preheat the oven to 350°F. Spray a 9 × 13-inch baking dish with cooking spray.

2. Heat the oil in a medium nonstick skillet over medium-high heat. Add the onion and cook, stirring occasionally, until it softens slightly, 2 minutes. Add the bell pepper and cook for 1 minute more. Stir in the garlic, cumin, chili powder, coriander, oregano, and salt, and cook for 30 seconds. Set aside to cool slightly.

3. In a large bowl combine the turkey, zucchini, eggs, oats, onion mixture, and ¼ cup of the tomato sauce. Mix with your hands until just combined, and then transfer to the baking dish and shape into a loaf about 5 inches wide and 2 inches high. Spoon the remaining tomato sauce over the top.

4. Bake until an instant-read meat thermometer registers 160°F, about 1 hour. Remove from the oven and let rest for 10 minutes before slicing.

Calories 260; Fat 13 g (Sat 3 g, Mono 5.1 g, Poly 3 g); Protein 23 g; Carb 11 g; Fiber 2 g; Chol 140 mg; Sodium 360 mg

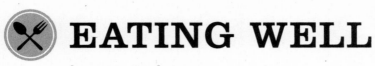

EATING WELL

keep it lean

This week's Eating Well focus is one of the most convincing cases for the power of small changes. Amazingly, you can lose more than six pounds a year by making this one simple change: choosing a lean meat over a high-fat one each day.

For example, if you have 3 ounces of skinless chicken breast for dinner instead of the same amount of T-bone steak, you save about 60 calories. That might not sound like a lot, but over the course of a year that adds up to 21,900 calories, which translates into a six-pound weight loss. The numbers are even more impressive when you consider that most people typically eat much more than 3 ounces of meat at dinner. After all, a typical restaurant-sized serving is about 10 ounces—or even more!

I know, I know: you probably already realize chicken breast is healthy and try to swap your red meat for white when you can. But if you feel like you are going to start clucking if you eat any more chicken, take heart. Chicken is only one of many lean-meat options you can include on your Usually list. You may be surprised at the variety of meats—even red meats—and poultry that make the low-fat grade. Give them a try and they can make healthy eating less of a bore and add more variety to your diet.

PROTEIN POWER Last week I talked about vegetarian sources of protein like nuts, seeds, beans, and legumes. When most people think of protein, though, they think of animal sources like beef, pork, and poultry, which, along with eggs, are our focus this week.

Protein (animal or vegetable) is an essential part of your diet, and critical to the health of every cell in your body. It helps build, repair, and maintain body tissue like muscle and is used to create red blood cells as well as to keep your hair, skin, and fingernails healthy. It's responsible for helping produce antibodies that fight off bacteria, viruses, and germs and keeps your immune system running strong—studies show that people low on protein are more likely to get sick than people who eat enough of this nutrient. Also, protein foods can be a boon to weight watchers because they tend to be among the most satisfying, making you feel full on fewer calories.

Most Americans get plenty of protein, but new research points to the possibility that many people over age 50 may not be getting enough. The Dietary Reference Intake for protein is 46 grams for women and 56 grams for men, but many experts contend that 70 to 90 grams of protein a day may be beneficial for older people, especially when it comes to maintaining healthy bones.

Research supports the health benefits of including more protein from vegetable sources (like beans, soy, nuts, and grains), as I discussed in Week 10, but animal sources (like meat, poultry, fish, eggs, and dairy) offer many benefits, too. The key is making sure you get your animal protein without too much saturated fat.

high-protein foods

FOOD	PROTEIN (IN GRAMS)
Meat, poultry, and fish (3 ounces cooked)	20–30
Yogurt, Greek-style low-fat (6 ounces)	17
Cottage cheese, low-fat (½ cup)	14
Tofu, firm (½ cup)	10–20
Yogurt, regular low-fat (6 ounces)	9
Milk, low-fat (1 cup)	8
Peanut butter (2 tablespoons)	8
Beans, cooked (½ cup)	7
Egg, hard-boiled (1 egg)	6
Pasta, cooked (½ cup)	3
Bread (1 slice)	3

RED DOESN'T ALWAYS MEAN STOP One of the most nutrient-dense sources of protein is red meat, but it's often blamed for much of the chronic illness and expanding waistlines in this country. It is true that most cuts of red meat, including beef, pork, and lamb, are laden with saturated fat and calories—major contributors to heart disease, obesity, and other problems. And as a whole, we eat far too much of it, from burgers and ribs to steaks and chops.

Most people would be better off getting less protein from animal sources and more from vegetable sources and fish, as you have been doing in recent weeks. But, to its credit, red meat is also full of key nutrients: zinc, iron, selenium, magnesium, and B vitamins. When you choose the leanest cuts, meat is actually quite a dietary bargain, giving you a wealth of nutrition per calorie.

Choosing lean cuts of red meat is easier than you might think. One easy rule of thumb is that the leanest cuts of pork and beef tend to have "loin" or "round" in the name. For example, beef top round, beef eye round, and pork tenderloin are the trimmest, coming remarkably close to skinless chicken breast in leanness. As you'll see in the chart on pages 260–261, other cuts of beef, pork, and some cuts of lamb are also reasonably low-fat choices.

The first step is to start with a lean cut of meat, but there are other things you can do to make your meal even slimmer. First, choose a "select" grade of meat—that means less fat is marbled throughout the flesh than in "choice" and "prime" grades. Then, trim off all visible fat, and use a cooking method that doesn't add extra fat to the dish—in fact, one that allows excess fat from the meat to drip off during cooking, like broiling, grilling, or roasting on a rack.

THE "SKINNY" ON GROUND BEEF When buying ground beef, don't be fooled by labels boasting "85% lean." That percentage may sound good, but it is actually very high in fat. The packagers are talking about percent lean by *weight,* not by calories. Meat that has a label of "85% lean" gets about half its calories from fat. Only ground beef that is 90% lean or higher qualifies as a Usually food.

You can eliminate about two-thirds of the fat in ground beef with this drain-and-blot method: after browning the meat, drain the fat from the pan, transfer the meat to a plate lined with paper towels, and blot the top of the meat with more paper towels.

GETTING WILD Most of us grew up on domestic meat sources like beef, pork, and lamb, but more "wild" meats like venison, buffalo, and elk are being eaten today. These meats are incredibly lean and are available, more and more, in markets around the country as well as in many restaurants. Some game has less fat than skinless chicken breast, yet like beef, game meats offer high levels of zinc, iron, and other nutrients, as well as protein.

Because this meat is so lean, game steaks are best served medium rare or rare. Don't overcook them or they will be tough. However, stew cuts of game are delicious slow-cooked or in a chili. Game can be an expensive treat if you are not lucky enough to know a hunter for your supply; but if you like it, it's well worth the cost. And with the growing popularity of game meats, you may find a reasonably priced buffalo burger at your local diner! Try one next time.

POULTRY PICKS Poultry such as chicken and turkey are mainstays of a healthy eater's repertoire. Even face-to-face with the most fattening menu, you can usually do okay with a grilled chicken or turkey sandwich. (Just be careful of the fat-laden toppings like cheese, mayonnaise, and salad dressing.)

However, not all poultry is as lean as it is made out to be. Sure, skinless chicken breast and turkey breast are the best in low-cal, high-quality protein. But if you grab a piece of roasted chicken with skin, you could be getting more fat than if you had a steak. You might opt for a turkey burger thinking it is a wise choice, but if the turkey is ground with dark meat and skin, as it is in most restaurants, you wind up with 10 times the fat you bargained for. So make sure you remove the skin from your poultry, and specifically ask your butcher for lean ground turkey. When cooking, bake, broil, poach, steam, or stir-fry, but keep your bird out of the fryer and away from the gravy, both of which pack on calories and unhealthy fats.

While sometimes overlooked by chicken and turkey fans, game birds are extremely lean and often look and taste like red meat. Ostrich, pheasant, quail, and squab are delicious and healthy and can make for a very special dinner. Choose wild duck, which has only half the fat of domestic duck. Domestic duck and goose are the fattiest of birds, so they should appear on your plate only rarely.

AN EGG-CELLENT FOOD When it comes to protein, don't overlook eggs, one of the most convenient, inexpensive, nutritious sources of high-quality protein around. They are low in calories and fat while being rich in B vitamins, vitamins D, E, and A, and choline. They also contain lutein and zeaxanthin, antioxidants that help maintain healthy eyes. They are easy to keep on hand and can be whipped up (literally!) in minutes. But because eggs are high in cholesterol (one large egg has 186 milligrams of cholesterol, more than half of the 300 milligrams daily limit recommended by the American Heart Association), they have been stuck on the nutritional hit list for the past twenty years.

It turns out eggs have been unfairly maligned. We now know the cholesterol you eat is not the main factor influencing your blood cholesterol. Trans and saturated fats are the culprits. So while you want to keep an eye on your cholesterol consumption to be on the safe side, it is far more important to focus on watching your intake of undesirable fats. Since an egg has just 5 grams of fat (1.5 grams of it saturated), one whole egg a day can fit neatly into a healthy diet.

But people often tend to eat two eggs at a time, which means 10 grams of fat, even cooked without butter. That's close to the amount of fat in that T-bone steak you are supposed to be trading in. And remember, you also have to count the eggs that are in baked goods and other recipes toward your one-egg-a-day limit.

To do eggs right, eat just one—a hard-boiled egg makes an energizing snack or breakfast on the run with a piece of fruit, for instance. You could also stick with egg whites, since all an egg's fat and cholesterol is found in the yolk. But as luck would have it, most of an egg's nutrients are in the yolk, too, so it is a trade-off. I like to split the difference, making my scrambled eggs with one whole egg and one egg white. This compromise works well with many egg-based recipes, too, and should help you keep to the suggested maximum of one whole egg a day.

fat and calories in meat and poultry

FOOD (3 ounces cooked, trimmed)	TOTAL FAT (G)	CALORIES	SATURATED FAT (G)	CHOLESTEROL	U/S/R
Beef					
Eye of round	3.5	138	1.2	63	U
Top sirloin	4.9	156	1.9	70	U
Top loin (strip) steak	5.4	155	2.1	67	U
Ground, 95% lean	5.6	145	2.5	65	U
Top round	4.3	169	1.5	76	S
Brisket, flat half	5.9	174	2.3	85	S
Flank steak	6.3	158	2.6	66	S
Chuck shoulder pot roast	6.6	167	2.2	83	S
Tenderloin	6.7	164	2.5	69	S
T-bone steak	7.4	161	2.6	47	S
Ground, 85% lean	13.2	212	5.0	76	R
Prime rib	17	247	6.7	82	R
Pork					
Ham, extra-lean	4.7	123	1.5	45	U
Tenderloin	5.4	159	1.9	80	U
Loin chop, center cut, lean	7.1	158	2.4	56	U
Ham, regular	7.7	151	2.7	50	S
Shoulder	11.2	198	4.3	85	R
Lamb					
Leg, shank	6.6	162	2.3	76	S
Shoulder	7.7	170	2.9	78	S
Leg, sirloin	7.8	173	2.8	78	S

*U = usually; S = sometimes; R = rarely

FOOD (3 ounces cooked, trimmed)	TOTAL FAT (G)	CALORIES	SATURATED FAT (G)	CHOLESTEROL	U/S/R
Game meat					
Elk	1.6	124	.6	62	U
Buffalo	2.1	122	.8	70	U
Venison (deer)	2.7	134	1.1	95	U
Poultry					
Egg whites (2)	0.1	34	0	0	U
Turkey breast, skinless	0.6	115	.2	71	U
Turkey, ground, extra-lean	2.3	128	0.6	60	U
Turkey breast, with skin	2.7	130	.7	76	U
Chicken breast, skinless	3.0	140	.9	72	U
Egg (1 whole)	4.8	72	1.6	186	S
Chicken breast, with skin	6.6	167	1.9	71	S
Chicken thigh, skinless	7.0	150	1.9	115	S
Chicken leg, with skin	7.6	156	2.1	108	S
Chicken thigh, with skin	12.6	195	3.5	115	R
Ground turkey, 85% lean	13.8	212	3.5	89	R
Domesticated duck, no skin	9.5	171	3.4	76	S

Too Much of a Good Thing?

If protein is so good for you, why not try one of the popular high-protein diets, which promise to help you shed pounds so quickly? First of all, too much protein—more than 150 grams a day—can tax your liver and kidneys. But that is not the biggest problem I have with the most extreme of these plans.

The real crux of these diets is that they strictly limit carbohydrates, and as a result ban or severely restrict some of the healthiest foods out there, foods like carrots, bananas, whole grains, and low-fat dairy products. Consequently, they can set you up for nutritional deficiencies and deny your body some of the most powerful disease-fighting foods available. In addition, some are over the top in saturated fat, which has long been linked with chronic disease.

One reason people lose weight so quickly on these plans is that when you severely restrict carbohydrates, your body has to access its glycogen, or stored glucose, for energy. As you deplete your glycogen stores, you also lose water—3 grams of water goes along with each gram of glycogen. That's why people lose so much "weight" immediately on a high-protein plan—as the body's glycogen stores are burned, you also lose a lot of water, which can put you at risk for dehydration and constipation.

Some more moderate high-protein plans (that allow the healthiest carbs and fats) are probably safe and can lead to sustained weight loss. But people tell me that these programs can get boring, and in the end, all that protein isn't the healthiest balance for a long-term eating plan.

HOW MUCH MEAT IS ENOUGH? Many diet books on the market today have meat as their centerpiece. But reams of research show that the healthiest diets aren't weighed down with lots of animal protein. Three to six ounces a day (with one egg or two egg whites counting as an ounce) is plenty. See page 291 for the amount of lean animal protein that best suits you.

action

Starting this week, choose meats, poultry, and eggs from the Usually and Sometimes lists (see pages 14–15), and keep servings to 3 to 6 ounces per day.

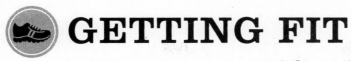

GETTING FIT

making exercise a lifestyle

Think about it. You spend only a small portion of time exercising. Even if you work out for an hour a day (which is much more than most people!), the other 23 hours a day are spent working, eating, sleeping, and performing all the other activities of daily life. By becoming more active during those 23 hours, you increase your fitness level and improve your health without even thinking about it.

MORE MOVEMENT, MORE BENEFITS Think about someone you know whose physical body and energy level you admire. It may be your neighbor with three children who works full-time and still finds time to go to the gym and coach soccer. Or maybe it's your coworker who puts in long hours and trains for marathons on the weekends. I'll bet that neither one of them spends much time on the couch watching television. They're active without thinking about it—and all that activity adds up to a healthier lifestyle.

While you can add movement to your life in a variety of ways, doing activities with your friends and family is one of the most enjoyable ways to become more active. I've talked before about the benefits of working out with a partner or buddy, and ways to encourage your kids to become more fit.

People who play sports like tennis, racquetball, and golf often play for the sheer enjoyment of the activity. Sure, they're getting in shape as they play, but the bottom line is that it's fun. Team sports like touch football, volleyball, and baseball are a great way to socialize and stay fit. Sign up for a league or set up a game with your family, friends, or neighbors. The emphasis may be on competition or just on having fun. Take another look at The Power of Play, page 129, for more fun-focused activities.

EVERYDAY ACTIVITY ADDS UP! Health experts recommend that most people get at least 30 minutes of moderate exercise every day. But activities like vacuuming, gardening, walking the dog, and climbing stairs can all count toward that total. Everything—from standing up out of a chair to walking down a hall to lifting weights or biking—counts, so try to increase physical activity in little ways throughout the day.

For example, park farther away from the store or take the stairs instead of the elevator when you're running errands or at work. Increase the intensity of whatever you do—even household chores like vacuuming, sweeping, and dusting can be challenging depending on how much effort you expend.

Remember, every bit of activity counts. In 20 minutes, an average 140-pound woman will burn approximately the following calories for these tasks (you'll expend more calories if you weigh more than 140 pounds, fewer if you weigh less).

Typing on a computer	36 calories
Cooking	58 calories
Gardening	70 to 100 calories
Dancing (moderate pace)	80 calories
Shopping	80 calories
Cleaning/housework	80 to 90 calories
Mowing grass with a push mower	90 calories
Walking (20:00/mile pace)	96 calories
Playing Frisbee	108 calories
Weight training	110 calories
Walking down stairs	120 calories
Walking (15:00/mile pace)	126 calories
Swimming	158 to 210 calories
Jogging (11:30/mile pace)	176 calories
Walking up stairs	350 calories

MOVE MORE AT WORK If you have a desk job, you can sneak in more activity. Even short exercise sessions will help strengthen your heart, burn calories, and tone your muscles. Brief breaks will stimulate your metabolism and give you a natural energy boost. Doing something physical stimulates your body and mind.

Walk away. Nothing beats a quick walk to clear your head—step outside for a change of scenery, or if the weather's bad, head for the stairs and walk up and down for a couple of minutes.

Take a dip. Sit in a stationary chair with your feet out in front of you. Gripping the edge of the chair and keeping your back straight, slowly lower your body 8 to 10 inches and then return to the original position; it will boost your heart rate and tone your shoulders and triceps.

Do it yourself. Run all your own errands. Every time you get up from your desk, you burn a few extra calories and keep your muscles in working order.

Take an Active Vacation

What's your dream vacation? Lying by the beach sipping a piña colada? Relaxation is great, but that doesn't mean you have to loll about all week. Look for ways to incorporate activity into your vacation and you'll feel better. In fact, active vacations are a growing trend. Some trips offer hiking, biking, or walking group tours; others allow you to kayak, raft, or trek.

Here are three great websites that focus on active vacations:

- **Backroads. www.backroads.com**
  Specializes in biking, walking, and multisport trips worldwide, and includes options for family adventures, singles trips, and private trips.

- **Adventures in Good Company. www.adventuresingood company.com**
  This company caters specifically to women looking for active and adventure vacations.

- **Mountain Travel Sobek. www.mtsobek.com**
  Mountain Travel Sobek offers more than 150 active vacations around the globe, and allows you to select your activity type and trip level.

Even if you decide not to opt for an active vacation, you can take time to hike through a new park when traveling. Nearly every city offers beautiful new vistas to explore. You're more likely to come home feeling refreshed if you include some physical activity during your trip.

Instead of taking one two-week vacation each year, consider breaking up your vacation time into shorter trips. According to one survey, more than two-thirds of all Americans say they need only one to three days to feel restored and relaxed. The majority say seeing new places, being away from work, and doing new or different things lead to a restful vacation, and more than half say exercising gives them energy on vacation.

So, plan to include activity on your next trip. You'll feel better, enjoy yourself more, and keep up your healthy habits on the road as well as at home.

Squeeze it. Keep a tennis ball or racquetball on your desk, and squeeze it as you talk on the phone—it will increase your hand, forearm, and grip strength and relieve tension, as well.

Shrug it off. One of the best ways to reduce neck and shoulder tightness is by performing simple shrugs. Stand up with your hands hanging at your sides and lift your shoulders as high as you can before returning to your original position. Repeat 10 times and then slowly lower your head toward your chest and take a deep breath.

Save gas. If you drive to work, leave your car five blocks away from your office and walk the difference. Then increase the distance for longer walking sessions. (If you take the train or bus, just get off at an earlier stop.)

Take the long way. When you head to the bathroom or for a cup of coffee, take the longest route possible—or add a few quick laps around the office before you return to your desk.

Tighten your tummy. When sitting at your desk, do a few chair crunches. Grasping the sides of your chair for balance, lift your legs and pull your knees toward your chest, and then slowly lower them back down. Keep your back straight as you do the crunches; as you become stronger, do them without holding the chair.

Be helpful. Volunteer to carry that heavy box into the office—just be careful not to strain your back. You'll burn a few extra calories and also maintain upper-body strength.

Take the stairs. Avoid the elevator whenever possible and opt for the stairs instead. If you work on the 30th floor, try getting off on the 25th floor instead. And if it's only a flight or two, the stairs are quicker than waiting for the elevator anyway.

action

Do one thing each day to increase the amount of activity you get in your daily life. That may mean parking a little farther from your office or taking more frequent stretch breaks at work.

 # FEELING GOOD

pampering

In the past weeks, you've become more mindful and begun to get in better touch with your inner spirit. But caring for the outside of your body—your physical self—can have positive and soothing effects on the mind and spirit, as well.

You already wash your face, brush your teeth, and perform other physical self-care tasks without thinking about them. Taking this a step further lets you care for and reconnect with your physical self. This might be as simple as taking a few minutes at night to moisturize your skin with a favorite lotion or signing up for a massage once a month.

Do you think spending money on yourself is frivolous or vain? Olivia, a 35-year-old child psychologist, used to feel that way. She never paid much attention to fashion or the way she looked, and felt that things like manicures and facials were self-indulgent luxuries. Throughout her adult life, Olivia focused her energy on intellectual pursuits. She graduated with her doctorate from a great school and had a thriving private practice in New York City. She gave all her energy and heart to the children she helped. But though her career was blossoming, she felt something was missing in her life.

Olivia realized that her life was out of balance. She spent so much time giving to and nurturing other people that she wound up feeling drained. While she was proud of her career accomplishments, she also realized that she didn't feel comfortable with her body. She'd never paid much attention to it, concentrating instead on her mind.

Olivia decided it was time to reconnect with her physical self. She pampered herself by indulging in regular manicures and pedicures. This seemingly small act has made her feel better about her physical appearance. She even carries herself differently and feels more confident and comfortable in her own skin.

"It's a way of treating my body like a valuable asset that I cherish," says Olivia. "It's like wearing nice underwear. Even if no one sees it, you feel special, and it reinforces that you are worthy of good things." Taking time to treat herself has helped Olivia find the balance between giving to others and replenishing by giving to herself.

RUB YOURSELF RELAXED Massage is more than a feel-good practice; hundreds of studies reveal that it has proven health benefits, too. Sure, you know that massage eases stress and encourages relaxation, but did you know it's used to treat conditions ranging from arthritis to migraines to high blood pressure?

In addition to reducing swelling, increasing blood flow, and improving circulation, massage helps prevent scar tissue from forming. It appears to improve immune function and stimulates lymph circulation. Regular massage can also improve muscular strength and reduce muscle spasms.

When you think of massage, you're probably thinking of what's called Swedish massage, but there are a variety of types to choose from. Here's the rundown on some of the most popular:

- **Deep tissue.** Deep tissue massage uses heavy finger pressure and usually is focused on one specific muscle group.

- **Reflexology.** This type of massage centers on the hands and feet. Practitioners use pressure on specific points that are believed to correspond to different organs of the body.

- **Rolfing.** Named after the person who created it, Rolfing is an extremely intense massage that involves stretching connective tissue.

- **Shiatsu.** Like reflexology, shiatsu massage involves the application of pressure to specific points of the body to restore energy, or "chi," to assist with healing.

- **Sports.** Sports massage is an umbrella term for massage that targets improved athletic performance, recovery, and/or injury prevention. It's similar to Swedish massage but often more intense.

- **Swedish.** Swedish massage is the most popular, and best-known, type in the United States. It employs a variety of strokes, including *effleurage*, or long, smooth strokes applied to the muscles.

- **Trager.** Named for the doctor who developed it, Trager massage involves shaking and rocking motions designed to release tension and loosen tight muscles.

- **Trigger-point.** Trigger-point massage involves the use of or pressure on specific areas of the body; the idea is to stimulate the trigger points to relax other muscle groups.

TREAT YOURSELF As our lives get more stressful, taking time to relax and slow down becomes even more important. Treating yourself to a massage, facial, manicure, haircut, or pedicure is a wonderful way to take some time to yourself—and improve your physical appearance and your mental outlook at the same time!

You don't need a fat wallet for a relaxing spa experience—you can do it yourself in less than an hour's time. Set out a few ingredients—candles, shampoo and conditioner, bath salts, relaxing music if desired, and thick, comfortable towels—so that you'll have everything you need. Let your kids and partner know that you're taking a "spa break" and will be unavailable—or, better yet, do it when you're home alone.

Light the candles and put on relaxing music. Run a warm bath with your favorite bath salts or essential oils and soak for at least 20 minutes. As you soak, you can apply a facial mask and deep-condition your hair. Close your eyes, listen to the music, and imagine all the tension flowing out of your body.

When you get out of the tub, picture your stressors draining away with the water. Afterward, take a few moments to rub your favorite lotion on your skin and dress in your favorite pajamas. Take a moment to feel how relaxed and at peace you feel—and for less than five dollars' worth of bath supplies!

action

This week, if you can, take time to pamper your physical body, even in a small way. Schedule a massage or a manicure, or simply take time to soak in a bath, or treat yourself to a new aftershave or cologne.

---

week 11 ACTION SUMMARY

- Shop to replenish your healthy pantry.
- Eat regular meals and snacks, stopping when you are at 7 on the Hunger Continuum (see page 61).
- Drink enough to stay well hydrated, including at least five glasses of water and a maximum of one sugary drink a day.
- Use healthy fats for cooking, dressings, and spreads.
- Eat two to four servings of fruit and three to six servings of vegetables each day.
- Check the ingredient list on your food labels.
- Get at least three servings of whole grains a day and limit refined grains.
- Eat fish at least twice this week.
- Eat at least one serving of nuts, seeds, beans, or soy each day.
- Record in your journal everything you eat and drink.

continues ›››

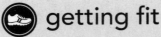 getting fit

- Walk for 20 to 40 minutes three times at mid- or high intensity.
- Stretch and do strength training and core training three times.
- Include a fun element in your fitness program.
- Do one thing to increase the activity in your everyday life.
- Continue to attend a fitness class.
- Note your activity in your journal.

feeling good

- Do the Five-Minute Breathing Exercise or take a minivacation once a day.
- Practice mindfulness.
- Say no to tasks you don't want to and don't have to do.
- Keep up your bedtime ritual.
- Do a deep relaxation or meditation exercise at least once.
- Optional:
  Tackle a clutter-clearing project.
  Explore journaling.
  Plan a special time with your partner or family.
  Reconnect with a friend.
  Do something to pamper your body.

WEIGHT

....

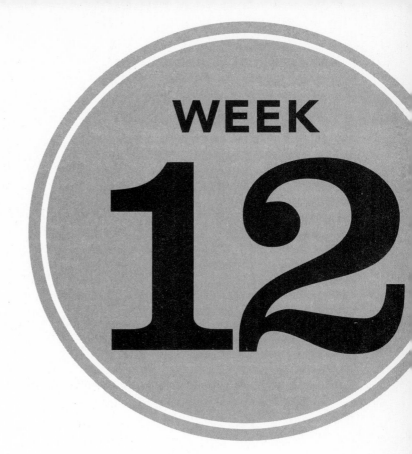

WEEK 12

this week's changes

1. Switch to low-fat dairy.
2. Sign up for a fitness event.
3. Donate some time to charity (optional).

this week's recipes
Say Cheese (and Other Dairy) Healthfully

- Pita Pizzas
- Buttermilk Mashed Potatoes
- Shells with Tomato Sauce and Ricotta
- Hot Cocoa
- Spinach-Feta Frittata

This week you'll learn how to make the smartest choices in the dairy aisle, from milk and yogurt to different types of cheeses. These recipes are mouthwatering examples of how to enjoy them easily and healthfully.

pita pizzas

SERVES 4 *These mini pizzas are perfect for lunch or a light dinner, and they are faster and healthier than pizza delivery. I used mushrooms as a topping here, but you can use fresh peppers, onions, olives, or any combination of vegetables. It's also a great way to use leftovers—try cooked broccoli or spinach.*

4 whole wheat pita breads
1 cup store-bought tomato sauce
1½ cups shredded part-skim mozzarella cheese
1 teaspoon dried oregano
2 cups sliced mushrooms

1. Preheat the oven to 400°F. Slice each pita all around the seam to make two rounds. Place the pita rounds, cut side up, onto baking sheets.

2. Spread 2 tablespoons pasta sauce on each round. Sprinkle with cheese and oregano, and top with mushroom slices. Bake for 10 to 12 minutes.

Calories 339; Fat 11.4 g (Sat 5 g, Mono 3.1 g, Poly 2 g); Protein 19.4 g; Carb 43.7 g; Fiber 6.1 g; Chol 25 mg; Sodium 846 mg

buttermilk mashed potatoes

SERVES 6 *Buttermilk gives these mashed potatoes a rich and creamy taste and an extra boost of calcium. No one will believe they are nearly fat free.*

2 pounds thin-skinned potatoes, such as Yukon gold (about 6 potatoes), unpeeled and cut into large chunks
1 cup low-fat buttermilk
Salt and freshly ground black pepper to taste

1. Place the potatoes in a medium pot, cover with water, and bring to a boil over a medium-high heat. Reduce the heat to medium and boil until the potatoes are tender, 15 to 20 minutes. Drain.

2. Put the buttermilk in a small saucepan and warm it slightly over a very low heat. Be careful not to let the buttermilk get hot, or it will curdle.

3. Mash the drained potatoes with a potato masher or fork, or use a hand mixer. Beat the warmed buttermilk into the potatoes with a wooden spoon. Season with salt and pepper to taste.

Calories 126; Fat .6 g (Sat .2 g, Mono .1 g, Poly 0 g); Protein 5 g; Carb 25.3 g; Fiber 2.7 g; Chol 2 mg; Sodium 47 mg

shells with tomato sauce and ricotta

SERVES 6 *This dish is pure comfort food to me, a favorite of my daughter's, and one I make regularly. The soft, creamy ricotta cheese mellows the acidity of the tomato sauce and adds a lovely texture, not to mention plenty of calcium and protein.*

1½ cups part-skim ricotta cheese
1 (28-ounce) can plum tomatoes with juice
1 tablespoon olive oil
2 garlic cloves, minced
¾ cup no-salt-added tomato puree or tomato sauce
¼ cup fresh basil leaves, chopped, plus some whole leaves for garnish
Salt and freshly ground black pepper to taste
1 pound whole grain shells, or other pasta

1. Bring a large pot of water to a boil. Take the ricotta out of the refrigerator to allow it to come to room temperature (not more than 30 minutes).

2. Put the plum tomatoes in a food processor or blender and pulse very briefly (about three times) until the tomatoes are finely chopped but not pureed.

3. In a large skillet, heat the oil over a medium heat. Add the garlic and cook until fragrant, about 1 minute. Add the chopped tomatoes and tomato puree and bring to a boil. Reduce heat to medium-low and simmer, stirring frequently, until slightly thickened, about 15 minutes. Stir in the chopped basil leaves and season with salt and pepper.

4. Meanwhile, cook the pasta according to the directions on the package. Drain and return to the pasta pot. Add the sauce and toss to combine. Divide the pasta among the serving bowls, top each with ¼ cup dollop of ricotta cheese and a basil leaf or two.

Calories 420; Fat 9 g (Sat 3.5 g, Mono 3.1 g, Poly .4 g); Protein 18 g; Carb 67 g; Fiber 10 g; Chol 20 mg; Sodium 490 mg

hot cocoa

SERVES 1 *This warming treat is a hundred times more delicious than the powdered, watery stuff you've been drinking. Plus, you get about a third of your daily requirement for calcium and all the antioxidants of real dark chocolate.*

1 cup plus 1 tablespoon nonfat milk, heated
2 teaspoons cocoa powder
2 teaspoons sugar

1. In a small saucepan, gently heat the milk, stirring, until just before a skin forms. Remove from the heat.

2. Mix the cocoa powder, sugar, and 1 tablespoon hot milk in a mug, and stir until it forms a paste. Add the rest of the hot milk and stir until mixed.

Calories 127; Fat .9 g (Sat .6 g, Mono .3 g, Poly 0 g); Protein 9.3 g; Carb 22.1 g; Fiber 1.1 g; Chol 5 mg; Sodium 132 mg

spinach-feta frittata

SERVES 4 *The combination of whole eggs and egg whites makes this frittata rich while keeping it lean. Feta cheese naturally has about a third less fat than other cheeses and adds big flavor.*

- 4 large eggs
- 4 egg whites
- 2 teaspoons olive oil
- 1 medium onion, chopped
- 1 (10-ounce) package frozen spinach, thawed and drained of excess water
- ¼ teaspoon salt
- ½ teaspoon freshly ground black pepper
- ¼ cup feta cheese, crumbled

1. In a medium bowl, whisk together the eggs and egg whites and set aside.

2. In a large ovenproof, nonstick skillet, heat the oil over a medium flame. Add the onion and sauté until it begins to soften, about 5 minutes. Add the spinach and heat for 1 to 2 minutes. Stir in the salt and pepper. Pour the egg mixture over the vegetables in the skillet, covering them evenly.

3. Reduce the heat to medium-low, cover, and let simmer until the egg mixture has set around the edges but is still somewhat liquid in the center, about 8 minutes. Sprinkle with the feta cheese.

4. Meanwhile, preheat the broiler. Place the skillet under the broiler, about 2 inches from the heat source, until the surface is set and golden brown, 1 to 2 minutes. Be careful not to overcook, or the egg mixture will become tough.

5. Cut the frittata into 8 wedges and serve.

Calories 148; Fat 7.9 g (Sat 2.2 g, Mono 3.7 g, Poly 1.0 g); Protein 12.5 g; Carb 7.3 g; Fiber 2.8 g; Chol 214 mg; Sodium 336 mg

EATING WELL

dairy done right

Chances are you grew up drinking milk—on your cereal, at lunch, and a tall glass at dinner. All that milk added up to lots of calcium for growing bones, but did you know that a seemingly innocent glass of whole milk has the same amount of fat as two pats of butter? A piece of cheese the size of your thumb contains the same amount, and a meager ½ cup of premium ice cream has the equivalent of almost four pats! If you pour whole milk on your cereal, indulge in ice cream regularly, or love to have cheese on everything, you are probably eating more butterfat than you realize. Welcome to Week 12, because now, as your final Eating Well change, it is time to skim the fat and switch to low-fat dairy.

When you see the results, you'll be glad you did. Each time you substitute a glass of 1% low-fat milk for a glass of whole milk, you save about 50 calories (and more than 4 grams of saturated fat). Over the course of a year, that adds up to a five-pound weight loss. If you take it a step further and nix the cheese on your daily sandwich, you save another 100 calories and drop another 10 pounds by the end of the year. In case you haven't noticed, between last week's changes and the changes I just mentioned, you could be 20 pounds lighter this time next year—without suffering, dieting, or depriving yourself. And your arteries will thank you, too.

LOW FAT, HIGH POWER Let's get our terms straight here. When I say *low-fat dairy*, I mean milk or yogurt that is either 1% or fat free (also known as nonfat or skim) and lower-fat cheeses like part-skim mozzarella, part-skim ricotta, and low-fat cottage cheese. I find those soft cheeses just as good in their reduced-fat form, but I generally avoid the nonfat varieties, because they simply don't taste good to me and/or have a lot of artificial ingredients. Low-fat buttermilk makes the skinny list, too. Despite its buttery name, it's not made with butter. Rather, it is thick, tangy cultured milk (it is made using the same kind of active cultures that are used to make yogurt. See Probiotics: The Good Bugs, page 280), and it's delicious for baking and in dressings.

As for other cheeses like cheddar, bleu, Parmesan, feta, and such, I find that only the full-fat "real thing" will do taste-wise. And because their flavor is so intense, a little goes a long way. So for those, I keep them in the Rarely category and sprinkle them sparingly, in small amounts, for maximum impact.

When you cut the fat from dairy, you wind up with a great nutritional bargain—low-fat milk products retain the wealth of nutrients of their full-fat counterparts.

Dairy is an excellent source of protein and the main source of riboflavin (an essential B vitamin), vitamin D, and calcium in our diets. When you go low-fat, you get all that without a lot of calories. Plus, dairy foods are satisfying and incredibly convenient. There is nothing easier than grabbing a yogurt, pouring some milk on whole-grain cereal, or munching some low-fat cheese and a piece of fruit for a healthy breakfast or snack. Or you could even buy a drinkable yogurt smoothie, a nutritious food you only need one hand to eat!

calcium-rich foods

FOOD	AMOUNT	CALCIUM (MG)
Calcium-fortified cereal	¾ cup	200–1000
Yogurt, regular, low-fat, plain	1 cup	448
Calcium-fortified orange juice	1 cup	350
Milk, low-fat	1 cup	300
Soy milk, fortified	1 cup	300
Yogurt, Greek-style, low-fat, plain	1 cup	265
Sardines	3 ounces	204
Tofu, processed with calcium	½ cup	204
Cheddar cheese, reduced fat	1 ounce	200
Salmon, canned, with bones	3 ounces	181
Mozzarella cheese, part skim	1 ounce	180
Sesame seeds	2 tablespoons	178
Soybeans, cooked	½ cup	130
Almonds	⅓ cup	110
Bok choy, cooked	½ cup	79
Cottage cheese	½ cup	69
Beans, cooked	½ cup	25–65
Oranges	1 medium	52
Kale, cooked	½ cup	47
Broccoli, cooked	½ cup	36

THE CALCIUM CONNECTION When most people think "dairy," they think "calcium," and for good reason. One cup of low-fat milk provides 300 milligrams of the mineral, about a third of the 1000–1,200 milligrams recommended each day. Calcium is an essential nutrient that gives structure and strength to bones and teeth, helps muscles work properly, and has a number of other critical functions. Most of the calcium in our bodies is stored in our bones, which act like a bank, saving and withdrawing the mineral as needed. Your bones have stored almost all they can by the time you reach 20 years of age (that's why consuming dairy products is so important to children and teenagers), although you can still make deposits through your 30s. After that, your goal is to maintain the calcium stores you have accrued to keep your bones strong. If you don't consume enough calcium, your bones must tap their reserves so that there are adequate amounts of the mineral in your bloodstream. Over time, this constant withdrawal weakens the bone and can lead to osteoporosis.

Is Greek Yogurt Better?

I have long been a fan of Greek-style yogurt and had been making it myself from regular yogurt for years before it became so widely available in stores. Greek yogurt is basically just regular yogurt that has been strained of much of its liquid (called whey), making it thicker and creamier with less tanginess than regular yogurt. It is wonderful as a snack with fruit and honey and ideal as a base for dips and spreads.

The straining process concentrates the protein in the yogurt but eliminates much of the naturally occurring sugar (lactose) and some of the calcium. So, while Greek yogurt gets a lot of press for being high in protein and low in sugar, it also has about a third less calcium. The bottom line: both low-fat Greek-style and regular yogurt are wonderful options. Each offers its own unique taste, texture, and nutrient benefits.

Calcium isn't the only factor in bone health. Exercise, like the walking and strength training you have been doing, is essential for building and maintaining bone, as are vitamin D, vitamin K, and vitamin C. Remember, though, that while getting enough calcium has many benefits (and most of us don't get enough), it is also possible to get too much, especially with all the calcium-fortified foods available now. More than 2,500 milligrams of calcium a day can lead to kidney stones and other problems. If you top off a few servings of dairy with a calcium-fortified cereal and calcium-fortified juice, you may be overdoing it.

LACTOSE INTOLERANCE For all its benefits, dairy is not good for everyone. Between 30 and 50 million Americans suffer from lactose intolerance, which means their bodies don't produce enough lactase, the enzyme needed to digest lactose, the sugar in milk. Lactose intolerance produces symptoms including cramps, bloating, gas, diarrhea, and nausea after the eating of dairy products.

However, many people with lactose intolerance have some ability to digest dairy products and can comfortably eat small amounts of milk or foods like hard cheeses and yogurt, which are naturally low in lactose. Lactose-free and lactose-reduced milks and lactase enzyme tablets are also available. If you suspect you are lactose intolerant, be sure to see your doctor for confirmation.

PROBIOTICS: THE GOOD BUGS You may have heard about the active cultures in yogurt or noticed "contains active cultures" on the label. Those cultures are actually good bacteria called probiotics. Probiotics, what I like to call good bugs, help maintain a healthy intestinal tract by warding off the bacteria that make us ill.

10 Ways to Bone Up on Calcium

Want to get more calcium into your diet? While you can always take a calcium supplement, there are a variety of simple ways to increase your daily intake of this important mineral:

1. Cook your oatmeal with low-fat milk instead of water.
2. Get a nonfat latte instead of a plain cup of coffee.
3. Make your hot chocolate with low-fat milk instead of water.
4. Sprinkle sesame seeds on your cooked rice, on salads, or in stir-fries.
5. Dollop plain, nonfat yogurt instead of sour cream on your baked potato.
6. Dip your vegetables in plain, nonfat Greek yogurt flavored with garlic and herbs.
7. Have a handful of almonds and an orange as an afternoon snack.
8. Top your salad with cubes of marinated tofu.
9. Treat yourself to a glass of vanilla-, strawberry-, or chocolate-flavored low-fat milk.
10. Toss a few handfuls of chopped kale, cabbage, or other dark leafy green in your next pot of soup.

Probiotics may also protect against gastrointestinal infections, boost the immune system, and even guard against some cancers.

Yogurt is the most common source of probiotics, but not all yogurts have them. Look for brands that boast "live and active cultures" on their label and look for the names of different probiotic cultures, like *L. acidophilus, L. bifidus, S. thermophilus,* and *L. bulgaricus* on the ingredient list. Also keep an eye out for other products that are now being spiked with probiotics, including cottage cheese and smoothies. They can help your digestive tract function at its best and may keep you healthy, as well!

THERE'S MORE THAN ONE WAY TO GET YOUR CALCIUM Whether you're lactose intolerant or not, dairy is far from the only way to get your calcium. There are many other calcium-rich foods to choose from, such as kale, bok choy (Chinese cabbage), broccoli, sardines, tofu, nuts, and seeds, plus an array of calcium-fortified foods including juices, cereals, and soy milk. See the chart on page 278 for the calcium content of different foods.

action
Eat two or three servings of low-fat dairy and/or other high-calcium foods each day.

GETTING FIT
competing against yourself
By now, in this last week of the program, fitness has become a healthy habit. Others around you may have noticed a difference in the way you look, while you've noticed how much better you feel. Maybe you have more energy, or you sleep more soundly, or you're able to get more done in the day. This week you'll discover how entering a fitness event can add a new spark to your regular routine.

TEST YOUR METTLE So, ready for a new challenge? Try signing up for a fitness event like a 5K walk or run. Nearly every community offers a slew of events, especially during the summer. Participating in one is a great way to stay motivated and test your fitness in a fun way.

You say you're not competitive? You don't need to be. Most of the people at fitness events don't stand a chance of winning—they're only competing against themselves. They may have registered to support a cause they believe in (many events are fund-raisers for charities or nonprofit organizations), or they simply wanted to participate in a community event.

Check the local papers for upcoming events or ask at your local health club or running store—they'll often have flyers and information about fitness events. Choose one that's close to home and that's a reasonable distance for you to cover. Races of 5K (3.1 miles) and 10K (6.2 miles) are popular, and at this point, walking three miles should be no problem. Write the date on your calendar and let people know you'll be participating—there's nothing more motivating than seeing people you know (and hearing them cheer for you!) when you're out on the course.

Consider asking a friend to participate with you—if you can train ahead of time, all the better. Having someone along will also help keep you from feeling nervous when you line up at the starting line. Selecting an event that raises money for charity is a way to do something good for the community and for your physical health at the same time.

Dee Sanders never imagined that she would become a marathon walker. Dee, 52, had been very close to her mother-in-law and was heartbroken when she lost her to leukemia. After her mother-in-law's death, Dee received information cards in the mail about an annual marathon to benefit the Leukemia & Lymphoma Society. She tossed the cards away because, although she was quite fit, walking 3 miles three or four times a week, she couldn't imagine running 26 miles!

Then a friend contacted her. He had cancer and was walking the marathon with his wife, and he encouraged Dee to sign up. Dee hadn't realized that many people walk the race. While 26 miles of walking still seemed like a lot, she felt that she could meet the challenge, especially with the inspiration of her friend and her mother-in-law's spirit to guide her.

The Leukemia & Lymphoma Society Team-in-Training Marathon for Walkers and Runners provided her with a coach and a four-month training plan. Dee successfully finished the marathon and raised thousands of dollars for the charity. "Once I crossed that finish line, I felt I could do anything," she said.

Since then, Dee has walked three more marathons with her 33-year-old daughter, Tracy. Each time, they've crossed the finish line holding hands. "It brought us really close—even closer than before," Dee says. Today she's a volunteer marathon coach, training and motivating other walkers. Her experience has changed her physically and spiritually. "I gained strength and endurance and improved my self-esteem," she says. "I've met the most positive, motivated, wonderful people, and it makes me feel good I am doing something to help."

Dee encourages everyone she meets to sign up for a charitable walk or other event. "You just have to experience crossing that finish line," she says. "You will never be the same again."

FROM WALKER TO PARTICIPANT If you have decided to take the plunge and enter an event, congrats! You may be surprised at how much fun you have. While you should be able to walk a 5K at this point, you can push yourself a little bit more by training to jog or run one. Like Dee, you may want to turn it into a fund-raising event, as well; visit www.active.com to look for events in your area. The 5K is the most popular distance, in part because most people can complete this distance.

You already know about the importance of comfortable, supportive walking shoes. If your shoes are in good shape, no problem; if they feel like they're wearing out, though, invest in a new pair. Running is much harder on your feet than walking is, and wearing the right shoes can prevent soreness and injury.

If you haven't added jogging or running to your walks, start out gradually, warming up for about five minutes. Then run for a minute or two, and when you tire, walk again. If you're huffing and puffing, you're going too fast, so use the talk test or check your heart rate monitor if you wear one to measure your effort. Run at a pace that's comfortable for you. As you become fitter, you'll naturally spend more of your "walk" running, and running will feel easier.

It's usually more convenient to register for the race before the big day—you can pick up your race number and packet the day of the event. Give yourself extra time to find a parking place, and visit the bathrooms. Take a few minutes to stretch and warm up before the gun goes off. If you feel a little nervous, try to enjoy the sense of anticipation.

Start off at a comfortable pace. It's natural to be excited, but try to relax and settle into your usual walking gait. You can always speed up later. Whether you walk or run, concentrate on your form, and on maintaining a good pace—you may wind up winning an age group award without even meaning to!

Afterward, take time to cool down, stretch, and rehydrate. Drink plenty of water and have a light snack if you're hungry. Talk to the people around you, or walk back to the finish line to cheer the competitors who are still finishing. (There will be someone behind you, I promise!) Savor the feeling of completing the race—you did it! Look how far you've come in less than three months.

GOALS ARE GOOD THINGS One of the reasons I recommend signing up for a fitness event is that it gives you a goal to train for. Research shows that people who set fitness goals are more likely to stick with their exercise routines and perform at a higher level than those who don't. That's one of the reasons at the beginning of this program I had you write down what improvements or changes you wanted to make in your life.

Just as important, setting goals also gives you a way to achieve successes along the way, and there's nothing more motivating than success. Research shows that achieving even relatively small goals develops your self-efficacy, or your belief in your own ability to accomplish a task. So, if you have small goals you're working toward on a daily, weekly, or monthly basis, and you achieve those goals, you feel confident, successful, and positive—and those positive feelings make it easier for you to achieve your "biggies," whatever those goals may be.

When you set a goal, like to participate in a local 5K walk or run, you have something specific to shoot for, and that can give your workouts new purpose. When you make a goal, consider where you are now—if you're already walking or jogging three miles pretty easily, a goal of running a 5K race a month or two from now is reasonable. Deciding to run a marathon three months from now is not.

As you're setting your goals, remember to make them specific and measurable. You may have heard of the acronym SMART, which is often used when goal-setting. SMART stands for:

- Specific
- Measurable
- Attainable
- Realistic
- Time-oriented

So, if you're going to run a 5K, your SMART goal to achieve that might be "I will run/walk for 30 minutes, three days a week, for the next four weeks until the race." The idea is to make your goal specific enough to measure and track your progress over time, as opposed to a more general goal like "I will run more often."

Finally, don't worry about how minor a goal may seem. By now you've learned that even a small goal—like, say, walking three times a week (hmmm, doesn't that sound familiar?)—can help keep you on target.

action

Find a fitness event to participate in and sign up for it.

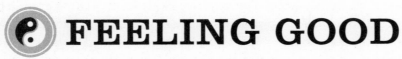

☯ FEELING GOOD

sharing the wealth

Throughout the preceding weeks, you've gotten in touch with yourself and strengthened the relationships with those closest to you—your family and friends.

This week, I encourage you to take that concern one step further and consider volunteering.

As a volunteer, you can participate in your community, create new friendships, and improve the quality of the place where you live and the lives of others. Yet volunteering doesn't have only external benefits—it's internally gratifying, as well. Anyone who has committed time or resources toward a good cause knows the satisfaction and the pleasure such work provides. Studies show that volunteers have higher levels of self-esteem and life satisfaction than those who don't give their time and energy. They may even live longer.

Volunteering can also teach you new skills and introduce you to talents you didn't know you had. Some volunteers enjoy what they do so much that they wind up taking jobs in a similar field; others like the chance to do something different from their normal jobs. In either case, volunteering is a way of connecting with others and getting in touch with the satisfaction of feeling like you're making a positive difference in the world.

WHERE TO START Maybe you already have an organization in mind that you'd like to support. If you're not sure what you'd like to do, consider your interests. Are you good with kids? Volunteering at your local Y, Boys Clubs, or Girl Scouts is an option. Or consider after-school or in-school tutoring programs.

If you're handy with a hammer, Habitat for Humanity and other programs can use you to help build houses. If you have business or office skills, nearly any non-profit will welcome you with open arms. The key is to find an activity that you'll enjoy—volunteering should enhance your life.

The amount of time you volunteer will depend on what you want. Would you rather have a regular commitment, like delivering Meals on Wheels two mornings every month, or do something more sporadic? Some volunteer jobs—being a Big Brother or Big Sister, for example—require a time commitment; others are one-shot deals.

Still not sure what you might want to do? Think about why you want to volunteer and what benefits you hope to gain from the experience. What kinds of skills, knowledge, or abilities can you share? What are your greatest strengths? What do you like—and dislike—doing? Do you want to work with other people or by yourself? Would you rather do clerical work in an office or be out interacting with people? How much time are you willing to give? What times would be best for you? Choose something that fits your schedule, your skills, and your temperament.

GETTING GRATEFUL Volunteering has a surprising effect on people; it makes them more grateful for what they have in their lives. Taking the time to "count your

Go Online to Do Good

You need look no further than your computer for volunteer opportunities. Sites like www.serve.gov, www.getinvolved.gov, and www.volunteermatch.org let you search for organizations looking for help, so you can decide which ones seem to be a good fit for your interests, time, and abilities.

blessings" may do more than just make you more aware of how fortunate you are—it may make you healthier, too. Experts studying gratitude are finding that experiencing gratitude can produce physical and emotional benefits.

While we tend to think of gratitude as thanking someone, it's more than that. Psychologists describe gratitude as a two-part process. The first part is acknowledging the goodness in your life; the second part is acknowledging that the source of this goodness isn't you. In other words, you might express gratitude to a higher power, to other people, or even to an animal, but you can't be truly grateful to yourself.

Recent studies found that people who listed things they were grateful for each week felt better about their lives, were more optimistic, slept better, and even got fewer colds than those who didn't pay attention to the good things in their lives. Other studies have found that people who experience greater levels of gratitude have higher levels of life satisfaction, even when they're faced with significant challenges. They're also better equipped to cope with the stressors of day-to-day life.

Yet most of us tend to focus on what we don't have (whether it's more money in the bank, a bigger house, time for an extended vacation) rather than what we do (good health, loving friends, happy kids). Fortunately you can learn to become more grateful—the more you practice, the easier it is.

In addition to volunteering, try these five ways to experience more gratitude in your daily life:

- **Put it in writing.** You can use your Food and Exercise Journal to list things you're grateful for, whether it's a beautiful spring day or your body's ability to walk for 30 minutes without getting winded.

- **Express yourself.** Write a letter to someone to thank him or her for making a difference to you—and mail it. You'll be amazed at the lift you get.

- **Thank a higher power.** If you pray or meditate, express gratitude for all you've been given—and for the ability to appreciate it.

- **Pass it around.** Families often go around the table at Thanksgiving and share something they're grateful for. Why not make it a tradition at your dinner table, as well?

action

This week's recommended action is to sign up to volunteer for one charitable project or event. Choose a one-time-only experience if you're nervous about committing to too much time at the outset—it can even be the fitness event.

week 12 ACTION SUMMARY

 eating well

- Shop to replenish your healthy pantry.
- Eat regular meals and snacks, stopping when you are at 7 on the Hunger Continuum (see page 61).
- Drink enough to stay well hydrated, including at least five glasses of water and a maximum of one sugary drink a day.
- Use healthy fats for cooking, dressings, and spreads.
- Eat two to four servings of fruit and three to six servings of vegetables each day.
- Check the ingredient list on your food labels.
- Get at least three servings of whole grains a day and limit refined grains.
- Eat fish at least twice this week.
- Eat at least one serving of nuts, seeds, beans, or soy each day.
- Get 3 to 6 ounces of lean animal protein a day.
- Get two to three servings of dairy or other high-calcium foods each day.
- Record in your journal everything you eat and drink.

continues ›››

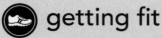

getting fit

- Walk for 20 minutes three times at mid- or high intensity.
- Stretch and do strength training and core training three times.
- Include a fun element in your fitness program.
- Do one thing to increase the activity in your everyday life.
- Continue to attend a fitness class.
- Sign up for a fitness event.
- Note your activity in your journal.

feeling good

- Do the Five-Minute Breathing Exercise or take a minivacation once a day.
- Practice mindfulness.
- Say no to tasks you don't want to and don't have to do.
- Keep up your bedtime ritual.
- Do a deep relaxation or meditation exercise.
- Optional:
  Tackle a clutter-clearing project.
  Explore journaling.
  Plan a special time with your partner or family.
  Reconnect with a friend.
  Do something to pamper your body.
  Donate some time to charity.

WEIGHT
....

you made it!

You did it! You've reached the end of the 12-Week Wellness Plan. Take a few minutes and retake the Lifestyle Questionnaire on page 25. I'm sure you'll score much higher on it this time around. Also, remeasure your chest, waist, and hips, and note your weight.

Looking at your numbers, and considering how you feel today, ask yourself whether you reached your goals. Where did you improve most? How much weight did you lose? Have you been surprised by how easy it has been to make small changes in your lifestyle—and how they've paid off? Or do you realize there are still some areas you need to improve?

the rest of your life (gulp!)

In some ways, the last 12 weeks have been the easy part. I've shown you how to make small, positive changes in the way you eat, move, and live and have given you the knowledge and template to incorporate those changes into your life. Now . . . you're on your own.

Oooh! Sounds scary, doesn't it? But here's the thing: you've learned a lot in just 12 weeks. You've learned the basics of good nutrition and how to eat to fuel your body and reach your optimal weight. You've discovered how to incorporate movement into your day and created a fitness program that you can maintain or step up to meet your goals. And you've learned how to reduce stress in your life and embrace a more fulfilling, happier lifestyle.

You did all that. I may have shown you the tools, but you put them into practice. Whenever you need to review any of these basic concepts, this book will be here, waiting for you.

STAYING MOTIVATED: A RELAPSE PLAN I'm sure there will be times when you find it more difficult to eat nutritiously, to find time to move your body, and to take time for yourself. How do you stay motivated over the long haul? By remembering that you needn't be perfect—every small step you take, every little improvement counts. If you go on vacation and your healthy eating plan goes out the window, pick it up again when you get back home. If work deadlines have kept you from exercising, start again next week. If you're feeling stressed, get back in the habit of doing the Five-Minute Breathing Exercise and taking time to decompress regularly.

Remember, at the halfway point, I discussed the importance of a backup plan. Etch this into your mind: it's always better to do something for your health—even something relatively minor—than to take no action at all.

If you've completely lost your motivation, however, and even your Plan B seems impossible, use this four-step relapse plan to get back on track:

1. **First, cut yourself some slack.** Don't call yourself names or beat yourself up because you've "failed." It's counterproductive and only makes you feel worse.

2. **Ask yourself why.** What's happening in your life to derail your progress? Is it work? Is it your family? Are you overeating to cope with stress, or do you feel overwhelmed by the thought of adding even one thing (say, walking) to your day? You have to understand why you're now struggling. Retaking the Lifestyle Questionnaire may help you address some of your current concerns.

3. **Remind yourself why you want to make positive changes.** You may want to spend some time journaling about this, or write a new letter to yourself about why it is important to you.

4. **Make a plan—and stick with it.** Even if you only say, "I'll walk for ten minutes after work tonight," that's better than doing nothing. If you've slacked off for weeks, you may want to start from Week 1—or you can jump back into the plan somewhere in the middle.

Some days, it's not easy—you will have times when your plate is filled with more Rarely foods than Usually ones. You will miss workouts. You will forget to take time to breathe, to relax, to meditate. But as long as you're improving over time, you're also on your way to becoming a fitter, healthier, happier you—all because you've made some small changes in your life.

Small changes really do add up.

appendix A how much should you eat?

First, determine how many calories you need by following these steps:

1. Multiply your weight (in pounds) by 15. This tells you the number of calories you need to maintain your weight. (This calculation assumes you are following the activities outlined in this book, or are otherwise moderately active.)

2. Subtract 500 from that number to lose one pound a week, or subtract 1,000 to lose two pounds a week. (Do not let your caloric intake fall below 1,200 calories per day, however.)

3. If you want to gain weight, add 500 to your maintenance calories.

If you weigh 150 pounds: That's 150 x 15 = 2,250 calories to maintain your weight and 2,250 – 500 = 1,750 to lose about a pound a week.

Then find the calorie range that you fall into in order to determine how many servings in each food group you should aim for per day. See Appendix C for serving amounts. Follow the Usually/Sometimes/Rarely food lists on pages 14–16 in making your food selections within each group.

FOOD GROUP	1,200–1,500 calories	1,500–1,800 calories	1,800–2,100 calories	2,100–2,600 calories	2,600–3,000 calories
Vegetables	3–4	4–5	5	5–6	6
Fruit	2	2–3	3	3–4	4
Grains and starchy vegetables	4–5	5–6	6–7	7–8	8–9
Meat, poultry, fish, and eggs	3–4 oz.	4–5 oz.	4–6 oz.	5–6 oz.	5–6 oz.
Nuts, seeds, beans, and soy	1	1–2	2	2	2–3
Dairy	2	2	2–3	2–3	3
Fats and oils	2–3	3	3–4	3–4	4

At the end of the 12-Week Wellness Plan, use your new weight to determine your new caloric needs and serving ranges.

appendix B sample week of healthy eating

Each day of this sample week adds up to about 1,500 calories. You can use this as a template, increasing or decreasing portions, or adding snacks, according to your caloric needs. Note that this week contains a healthy balance of Usually, Sometimes, and Rarely foods.

	DAY 1	DAY 2	DAY 3
BREAKFAST	Banana-walnut oatmeal (1 cup cooked oatmeal made with nonfat milk, with ½ banana and 3 tablespoons walnuts)	Cheerios (1½ cups) with nonfat milk (1 cup) and sliced strawberries (½ cup)	Strawberry Smoothie (PAGE 76)
SNACK	1 hard-boiled egg	Almonds (⅓ cup) and raisins (¼ cup)	Apple slices with peanut butter (1 apple with 1 tablespoon peanut butter)
LUNCH	Minestrone Soup (PAGE 55), with Parmesan cheese (1 tablespoon) and small green salad with Balsamic Vinaigrette (PAGE 117) (1 tablespoon)	Grilled chicken breast (4 ounces) over large mixed green salad with Balsamic Vinaigrette (PAGE 117)	Turkey sandwich (3 ounces turkey, lettuce, tomato, and avocado on a whole wheat roll), Vegetable soup (1 cup)
SNACK	Nonfat vanilla yogurt (1 cup)	Baby carrots (1 cup) dipped in Mustard-Dill Sauce (PAGE 117)	Cookies and milk (2 small chocolate chip cookies and 1 cup nonfat milk)
DINNER	Roast Pork Tenderloin (PAGE 248), Buttermilk Mashed Potatoes (PAGE 273), steamed broccoli, Poached Pears in Red Wine Sauce (PAGE 163)	Pita Pizzas (PAGE 272), Sorbet (½ cup)	Citrus-Ginger Flounder with Snow Peas (PAGE 209), brown rice (1 cup)

DAY 4	DAY 5	DAY 6	DAY 7
Banana–Peanut Butter Smoothie (PAGE 76)	Berries with yogurt, nuts, and honey (1 cup berries, 1 cup low-fat plain yogurt, ⅓ cup nuts, and 2 teaspoons honey)	Apple Crunch Oatmeal (PAGE 78)	Whole wheat English muffin with Creamy Honey Walnut Spread (1 tablespoon, PAGE 118)
1 peach	1 hard-boiled egg	Cheese and fruit (1 ounce Cheddar, 1 cup grapes)	Fresh fruit salad (1 cup) with nonfat vanilla yogurt and ¼ cup chopped nuts
Large spinach salad with mushrooms, tomatoes, chickpeas, chopped hard-boiled egg, and orange slices, with Citrus-Ginger Dressing (PAGE 116) and whole wheat pita bread	Middle Eastern Platter: Tabbouleh (PAGE 187), hummus, and ½ whole wheat pita with lettuce, tomato, and olives	Peanut butter and jelly sandwich (2 tablespoons peanut butter and 1 tablespoon jelly on whole wheat bread) and 1 orange	Lentil Soup (1 cup, PAGE 230) with whole-grain roll
Cheese and crackers (1½ ounces reduced-fat cheese with 5 whole-grain crackers)	Cantaloupe (½) and low-fat cottage cheese (½ cup)	Baby carrots (1 cup) dipped in hummus (2 tablespoons)	Hot Cocoa (1 cup, PAGE 275)
Burger and "Fries" [3-ounce turkey burger on a whole-grain bun with lettuce, tomato, onion, pickle, and ketchup, Baked Fries (PAGE 188)]	Linguini with Shrimp (PAGE 32) and sautéed spinach (1 cup)	Small green salad with olive oil (2 teaspoons) and vinegar and White Chili (PAGE 232)	Lemon Pepper Chicken (PAGE 31) with whole wheat couscous (½ cup) and Balsamic Swiss Chard (PAGE 137)

appendix C serving sizes

Remember, it is okay to have more than one (or less than one) "serving" of a food at a time. Just count it that way.

vegetables
(3 to 6 servings per day)
- ½ cup cooked or raw chopped vegetable
- 1 cup raw leafy vegetable
- 6 ounces (¾ cup) vegetable juice

fruits
(2 to 4 servings per day)
- 1 medium fruit: apple, orange, peach, pear, etc.
- ⅓ cantaloupe, honeydew, or other melon (1 cup cubed)
- ½ grapefruit
- ½ banana
- ½ cup canned fruit
- 1 cup fresh berries
- ¾ cup fruit juice
- ¼ cup dried fruit

grains and starchy vegetables
(4 to 9 servings per day)
- 1 slice bread
- ½ cup cooked grain (bulgur, oats, etc.), rice, or pasta
- ½ cup cooked hot cereal
- ¾ cup cold cereal
- ½ pita pocket
- 1 medium potato
- 1 small sweet potato or yam
- 1 ear corn or ½ cup corn

meat, fish, poultry, and eggs
(3 to 6 ounces per day)
- 1 ounce cooked meat, poultry, or fish
- 2 egg whites
- 1 whole egg

beans, soy, nuts, and seeds
(1 to 3 servings per day)
- ½ cup cooked beans, peas, or lentils
- ½ cup tofu, tempeh, or soy beans
- 1 cup soy milk
- ⅓ cup nuts
- ¼ cup seeds
- 2 tablespoons peanut butter or other nut butter

dairy
(2 to 3 servings per day)
- 1 cup milk
- 1 cup yogurt
- ½ cup cottage cheese
- 1½ ounces cheese

fats and oils
(2 to 4 servings per day)
- 2 teaspoons oil, margarine, butter, or mayonnaise
- 2 tablespoons regular dressing
- 4 tablespoons reduced-fat dressing

Use these visual aids to eyeball serving sizes:

THIS SERVING . . .	IS ABOUT THE SIZE OF . . .
3 ounces of meat, poultry, or fish	A smart phone
1 medium fruit	A baseball
½ cup cooked vegetables, fruit, pasta, rice, or other grain	Half a baseball
1 medium potato	A computer mouse
1 cup leafy greens	4 lettuce leaves
1½ ounces cheese	4 dice or 1 ice cube
2 tablespoons peanut butter	A golf ball
1 teaspoon fat	The tip of your thumb

appendix D supplement recommendations

Supplements cannot take the place of a good diet. We simply don't know enough about all the healthful properties of different foods and how they complement one another to put them into a pill. And there is not much evidence that there is any long-lasting benefit from taking them. Besides, I am not a big fan of pills. I don't think people should have to take a handful every day to stay healthy.

That said, a multivitamin and other supplements can be taken as a kind of insurance policy to fill in nutritional gaps. Some nutrients that Americans typically do not get enough of, which vitamins can cover, are vitamin D, folic acid, vitamin B12, iron, and calcium. Choosing the right "multi" can be a challenge. Many on the market are overloaded with some nutrients and skimp on others. Many also toss in a hodgepodge of herbs and other ingredients that are ineffective and expensive at best, and harmful at worst.

I recommend choosing a vitamin that provides 100% of the Daily Value for most nutrients, without any herbal extras. With some nutrients, you may be better off taking less than the Daily Value (iron, for example, if you are a man or a postmeno-pausal woman), and with some, you may want to take more for disease prevention (like vitamin D). Below and on the following page is a list of nutrients and amounts to consider when supplement shopping. It may be hard to find a supplement that fits your needs exactly, but you should be able to find an inexpensive brand that comes close. Of course, if you are pregnant, nursing, or have a medical condition, be sure to consult your doctor before taking any supplement.

NUTRIENT	DAILY VALUE	UPPER LIMIT	RECOMMENDED AMOUNT FOR A MULTIVITAMIN	COMMENTS
Vitamins				
A	5,000 IU	10,000 IU	3,000–5,000 IU	At least 20% should be from carotenoids.
C	60 mg	2,000 mg	75–200 mg	
D	400 IU	4,000 IU	600–800 IU	
E	30 IU	1,000 mg	30–100 IU	
K	80 mcg	n/a	80 mcg	
B_1 (Thiamin)	1.5 mg	n/a	1.5 mg	
B_2 (Riboflavin)	1.7 mg	n/a	1.7 mg	

continues ›››

NUTRIENT	DAILY VALUE	UPPER LIMIT	RECOMMENDED AMOUNT FOR A MULTIVITAMIN	COMMENTS
B$_3$ (Niacin)	20 mg	35 mg	20 mg	
B$_6$	2 mg	100 mg	2 mg	
Folic acid	400 mcg	1,000 mcg	400 mcg	
B$_{12}$	6 mcg	n/a	6–25 mcg	People over 50 should look for a multi with 25 mcg; others should look for 6 mcg.
Biotin	30 mcg	n/a	30 mcg	
Pantothenic	10 mg	n/a	10 mg acid	
Minerals				
Calcium	1,000 mg	2,500 mg	200–1,000 mg	Many multis have only 200 mg. Consider a separate calcium supplement to get 1,000 mg.
Iron	18 mg	45 mg	0–18 mg	Men and postmenopausal women should take a maximum of 10 mg iron.
Phosphorus	1,000 mg	4,000 mg	0–1,000 mg	Most of us get plenty of phosphorus, and too much can impair calcium absorption. The less in a supplement, the better.
Iodine	150 mcg	1,100 mcg	150 mcg	
Magnesium	400 mg	350 mg	100 mg	Most supplements contain no more than 100 mg. Consider a separate supplement for more, but do not exceed 350mg total from supplements.
Zinc	15 mg	40 mg	8–15 mg	
Selenium	70 mcg	400 mcg	70–100 mcg	
Copper	2 mg	10 mg	.9–2 mg	
Chromium	120 mcg	n/a	30–120 mcg	Choline, chloride, potassium, boron, manganese, molybdenum, nickel, silicon, and vanadium are often in multis and are safe at the Daily Value but not necessarily beneficial in supplement form.

appendix E resources

Visit my website **www.elliekrieger.com** to connect with me, get more recipes, watch videos, and read my blog and articles.

EATING WELL

Academy of Nutrition and Dietetics
The nation's largest organization of food and nutrition professionals. It provides solid nutrition information and can help you find a registered dietitian in your area.
www.eatright.org

Center for Science in the Public Interest
A nonprofit nutrition advocacy organization famous for uncovering food and nutrition issues that affect the public. It also provides useful information to consumers and sets the record straight on complex issues. It publishes the excellent *Nutrition Action Healthletter.*
www.cspinet.org

Choose My Plate Super Tracker
This website from the United States Department of Agriculture (USDA) has online tools that help you track the foods you eat and your physical activity as well as your weight management progress. It also lets you look up info for over 8,000 foods and compare foods side-by-side.
www.choosemyplate.gov/

Consumer Lab
This company objectively tests and evaluates nutrition supplements and other products and supplies the results to consumers.
www.consumerlab.com

Cooking Light
An excellent magazine that covers fitness and lifestyle as well as food and nutrition. The recipes are top-notch, and you can access many for free online. I also recommend their series of cookbooks.
www.cookinglight.com

CSAs (Community Supported Agriculture)
Find CSAs near you with this handy website.
www.localharvest.org

Eating Well
A food magazine with a wealth of high-quality, healthful recipes and insightful coverage of food and nutrition issues.
www.eatingwell.com

Fast Food Apps
These three iPhone apps let you calculate the calories in your fast food meal:

FAST FOOD CALORIES www.itunes.apple.com/us/app/fast-food-calories

FAST FOOD CALORIE COUNTER www.itunes.apple.com/us/app/fast-food-calorie-counter

NUTRITION FACTS www.itunes.apple.com/us/app/nutrition-facts

Fish consumption advisories
This website links you with local fish advisories nationwide.
www.epa.gov/ost/fish

Fit Day
This site includes an online diet journal and detailed nutrition information for thousands of foods.
www.fitday.com

Fooducate
One of my favorite apps for the iPhone, Fooducate lets you scan a label and tells what a food really contains. Great for shopping on the go.
www.fooducate.com

Healthfinder
A website developed by the U.S. Department of Health and Human Services as a resource for finding government and nonprofit health information on the Internet, it links to more than 1,700 health-related organizations.
www.healthfinder.gov

Local Harvest
This site is an excellent resource for finding sources of organically grown food ranging from restaurants to farmers' markets to CSAs.
www.localharvest.org

Melissa's World Variety Produce
Order organic and exotic fruits, vegetables, and other specialty foods online or find out where to get them in your area.
www.melissas.com

My Net Diary This free online food diary site lets you track the amount of calories you eat in a day. www.mynetdiary.com

Nutrition Data Here you can find detailed nutrition information and analysis tools to help you choose the healthiest foods. www.nutritiondata.com

Office of Dietary Supplements This website from the National Institutes of Health provides reliable, scientific information about dietary supplements. www.ods.od.nih.gov

Seattle's Finest Exotic Meats This company carries an amazing variety of different game meats and poultry. www.exoticmeats.com

Shop Natural A cooperatively run online health food store that offers a wide variety of groceries, from whole-grain cereals to nut butters to soy foods, to members in the Southwest. www.shopnatural.com

USDA Food and Nutrition Information Center This website gives you access to the National Agricultural Library and provides information about food composition and dietary guidelines. www.nal.usda.gov/fnic/

GETTING FIT

Active.com This site lets you search for active events by type of activity, distance, and location. www.active.com

American Council on Exercise The American Council on Exercise (ACE) is the largest nonprofit fitness certification and education provider in the world. They have numerous fitness publications and reliable information online. They can also help you find a certified trainer in your area. www.acefitness.org

American Volkssport Association A network of walking clubs and organizer of walking events nationwide. www.ava.org

Fit Click If you're bored with your exercise routine, check out this site for thousands of free exercise routines that will challenge mind and body. www.fitclick.com

Fitness Walking Logs You'll find a free walking log at these sites: www.the-fitness-walking-guide.com/walking-log.html www.realage.com/shape-up-slim-down/walking/5-ways-to-make-walking-a-habit

Full Fitness Looking for some new weight-training moves? This site includes exercises you can do with free weights, exercise bands, or weight machines. www.fullfitness.net

Heart Rate Monitors These three companies offer a variety of heart rate monitors, pedometers, and other fitness accessories: www.heartmonitors.com www.polarheartratemonitors.com www.cardiosport.com.

iBody Fit This site offers free online workouts that you can view online and on your TV and smartphone. www.ibodyfit.com

Map My Walk One of my favorite sites for walkers. You can create and measure your own walking routes or choose a route near your home or office. www.mapmywalk.com

Mayo Clinic Reliable, expert answers to common fitness questions www.mayoclinic.com/health/fitness/MY00396/TAB=expertanswers

Online Fitness Log Want to plan, track and personalize your exercise plan? You can do it on this motivating site. www.onlinefitnesslog.com

Online yoga You needn't leave the house to do yoga; this site offers free videos of different styles and levels of yoga that you can follow along with at home.

Road Runner Sports This catalog company offers running and walking shoes, gear, and accessories like heart rate monitors, pedometers, and body fat monitors. www.roadrunnersports.com

Title 9 Sports This company is geared toward active women. It sells athletic gear, swimsuits, underwear, shoes, sports bras, and accessories.
www.title9sports.com

The Walking Connection This website provides information, products, and services for walkers and hikers. Read articles, find out about walks and hikes in your area, and learn about exciting active vacations.
www.walkingconnection.com

The Walking Site This site includes message boards, motivation tips, and a list of local clubs you can join.
www.thewalkingsite.com

Wind Chill Heading out for a walk in the cold? Check the wind chill at this site first.
www.nws.noaa.gov/om/windchill

Workout Box This site lets you customize programs to meet your specific goals; you can also track your progress.
www.workoutbox.com/workouts

FEELING GOOD

Adventures in Good Company This company caters specifically to women looking for active and adventure vacations.
www.adventuresingoodcompany.com

The American Institute of Stress A nonprofit organization that provides information on all stress-related subjects. They have a large up-to-date library, and they can refer you to a professional.
www.stress.org

Backroads This company specializes in biking, walking, and multisport trips worldwide and includes options for family adventures, singles trips, and private trips.
www.backroads.com

Blogging Sites Want to set up your own free blog? Check out one of these three sites:
www.blogger.com
www.livejournal.com
www.opendiary.com

Craigslist This well-known site lets you list belongings you'd like to get rid of. It is also a good place to find used exercise equipment and even find fellow walkers or other fitness partners in your area.
www.craigslist.org

The Center for Mindfulness in Medicine, Health Care, and Society This part of the University of Massachusetts Medical School furthers the practice of mindfulness for individuals, institutions, and society. It also offers a stress-reduction program.
www.umassmed.edu/cfm

eBay Get rid of the things you no longer need or want—and get paid for them. You can also find good deals on exercise equipment you may need.
www.ebay.com

Freecycle Clutter can cause stress, and this unique site lets you get rid of yours. Offers household items, clothing, toys, and other goods for free to people in your community.
www.freecycle.org

Laughter Yoga Laughter Yoga by phone is free and occurs about 14 times a day for 15 to 20 minutes at a time.
www.laughteryogausa.com/laughteronthephone.html

The Meditation Society of America's Meditation Station Use this website to learn more about the benefits of meditation and explore different meditation techniques.
www.meditationsociety.com

Mountain Travel Sobek This company offers over 150 active vacations around the globe.
www.mtsobek.com

The National Sleep Foundation This nonprofit organization supports the study of sleep and sleep-related disorders. Its website includes helpful information for getting better-quality sleep.
www.SleepFoundation.org
www.myfreeyoga.com

Volunteer Opportunities These three sites allow you to search for organizations in need of volunteers:
www.getinvolved.gov
www.serve.gov
www.volunteermatch.org

acknowledgments

I am grateful to all the talented people who made this book not only possible but truly excellent. Thank you:

Kelly James-Enger, extraordinary coauthor, for being a true pro and for putting your heart into this.

Emily Takoudes, editor, for your vision in reimagining this book and your hard work bringing it to life.

Jane Dystel and Miriam Goderich, literary agents, for your unwavering support and guidance from the very beginning.

Robert Flutie and Hilary Polk-Williams, from Flutie Entertainment, for keeping the ship on course and helping the tide rise ever higher.

Melanie Acevedo, photographer; Cyd McDowell, food stylist; Sara Smart, prop stylist; Suzanne Katz, makeup artist; Ivonne Frowein, wardrobe stylist; Jane Treuhaft, art director; for creating such a beautiful cover shot.

Ashley Tucker, designer, who, remarkably, can take a simple Word document and turn it into an engaging, important tool that is a pleasure to read and put to use.

My treasured family and friends for believing in me and supporting me, always.

index